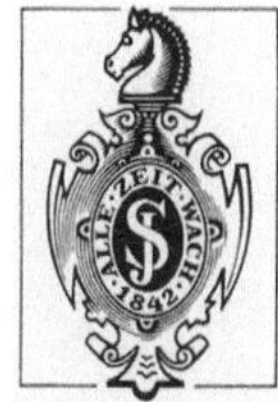

Knut Korth

Percutaneous Surgery of Kidney Stones

Techniques and Tactics

Foreword by W. Mauermayer

With 65 Figures and 3 Color Plates

Springer-Verlag
Berlin Heidelberg NewYork Tokyo 1984

Dr. med. Knut Korth
Loretto-Krankenhaus
Urologische Abteilung
Mercystr. 6–14
D-7800 Freiburg i. Brsg.

Translator

Virginia Sonntag-O'Brien

Belfortstr. 19
D-7800 Freiburg i. Brsg.

German edition
Perkutane Nierensteinchirurgie
© by Springer-Verlag Berlin Heidelberg 1984

Library of Congress Cataloging in Publication Data. Korth, Knut, 1936– Percutaneous surgery of kidney stones. Translation of: Perkutane Nierensteinchirurgie. Includes index. 1. Kidneys—Calculi—Surgery. I. Title. [DNLM: 1. Kidney Calculi—surgery. WJ 356 K85p]   RD575.K6713 1984   617'.461   84-10647
ISBN-13: 978-3-642-69849-1   e-ISBN-13: 978-3-642-69847-7
DOI: 10.1007/978-3-642-69847-7

Reproduction of figures: Gustav Dreher GmbH, Stuttgart

2122/3130-543210

Foreword

In recent years the treatment of kidney stones has taken on a new dimension, thanks to modern techniques. E. Schmiedt and Ch. Chaussy revolutionized the therapy of kidney stones with their extracorporeal shockwave lithotripsy. After percutaneous fistulization of the renal cavities by ultrasonically controlled puncture became a routine procedure, the obvious next step was to use the same approach, after dilating the track, to carry out intrarenal operations.

Dr. Knut Korth has been using this operative technique for some time now. He has gained a great deal of experience, having treated hundreds of patients who have come to him from all parts of Europe. In this book he describes the endoscopic technique which he has used in 400 cases. He does not attempt to compare and contrast his method with others, but rather describes and discusses the route *he* has taken. The book hence takes on a very subjective character – in the positive sense of the word. Dr. Korth believes – and emphasizes – that puncture should be performed by the urologist himself so that the final responsibility for an operation is not divided. Our own experience in exclusively urological operations without the help of a radiologist confirm this position.

Korth has developed many ideas – some in the form of instruments – for transcutaneous operations. He describes in detail the various procedures according to the type of stone, providing numerous examples.

As is always the case when new methods are introduced into surgery, those who are particularly experienced try to broaden the indication spectrum. The author has incorporated the opening of strictures at the ureteropelvic junction, the resection of papillary tumors, and the operation of renal cysts into the realm of percutaneous management. This is the right of a pioneer. Critical observation after a longer period of time will decide whether such ventures are justified.

The author has written this book with total commitment and "life-blood" but manages to keep a critical eye open. The book is full of personal ideas and experiences.

I wish this monograph on percutaneous surgery of the kidney much success and wide circulation.

Munich   Wolfgang Mauermayer

Preface

Although Goodwin performed the first puncture of the kidney as long ago as 1955, it was not until more than 20 years later that the percutaneous approach became a routine method (for example by Günther et al.). It was employed not only for emergency drainage of urine, but also for diagnostic procedures, for example the measurement of intrarenal pressure and the orthograde X-ray demonstration of obstructed urine flow. In 1976 Fernström removed kidney stones with a forceps through a percutaneous track. The first endoscopic stone operation was performed several years later (Smith, Alken). Ultrasound was first used in 1977 to disintegrate kidney stones via pre-existing drainage tracks (Kurth et al., Rathert et al.). In 1981, Marberger introduced the first percutaneous nephroscope for the ultrasonic disintegration of kidney stones, taking an instrument already used in the bladder and modifying it for the kidney. Since then, other instruments and percutaneous nephroscopes have been developed (Alken, Wickham, Korth), providing a broad spectrum of aids for this special type of endourology.

This volume is intended to serve as a practical handbook for the percutaneous surgical treatment of kidney stones, as performed in the urological department of the Loretto Hospital in Freiburg. It is based on the experience gained in operating on 400 patients. All of the operations were carried out by a *single* surgeon, who performed both the radiologic and sonographic parts of the percutaneous technique as well as the actual surgical treatment of the stones. The technique was applied for *every type* of kidney stone, which made it necessary to work out special procedures in particularly difficult cases, such as those involving staghorn calculi. Special attention is thus given to the complications that can arise during the percutaneous operation, including how to assess them and ways to avoid them.

Numerous practical tips and tricks which are essential for handling various situations are provided, but theoretical ballast is left out. The method is purposely not compared with extracorporeal shockwave lithotripsy or open surgical techniques.

Freiburg   Knut Korth

Contents

A. Introduction

The percutaneous management of kidney stones, in my opinion, signifies a revolution in kidney stone surgery. A large organ, which up till now could only be operated on by extensive surgical measures, can now be treated by endoscopic diagnostics and therapy. Just a few years ago this was unthinkable. Further sophistication of the surgical instruments will allow diagnosis and therapy to be carried out on the kidney the way they have been performed on the bladder. First, that means that the kidney will no longer be surgically exposed as, for example, in making differential diagnoses of non-calcified stones or papillary renal tumors. Suspicion of tuberculosis will no longer be clarified by time-consuming investigations, as the percutaneous approach will make it possible to provide sample excisions for histologic diagnosis. It will no longer be necessary to use a 20 cm incision to remove a small ureteral stone or a simple renal stone. Large stones can also be removed by the percutaneous technique, although in some cases several sessions may be necessary.

Particularly with regard to kidney stones, the percutaneous method demands that all surgical thinking be turned around. A kidney which has previously been operated on must no longer be the dread of the surgeon, who usually equates a third kidney operation with a nephrectomy. On the contrary, the scars left from the previous opera- in that case provide protection for the kidney. They surround the sensitive organ with a thick callus and thus protect the kidney from unintended perforations, for example, which can occur during kidney stone disintegration. The scars fix the kidney at the lateral abdominal wall, preventing the percutaneous track from being cut off by respiratory movements. The firm tissue of these scars provides for a very stable access track into the kidney after 1 to 2 days. Furthermore, scar tissue cuts off many tiny sensitive nerve branches, allowing even thick, hard scar calluses to be painlessly penetrated and dilated.

Percutaneous kidney stone surgery makes it possible for the first time to operate on older and poor risk patients, particularly since it can be carried out under local anesthesia.

One of the most important factors of kidney stone surgery loses its significance under the percutaneous technique: it is no longer necessary that the kidney be free of stones at the end of the operation. Should the operation prove to be too lengthy or if there is too much bleeding, it can be discontinued at any time. The instrument is removed and a nephrostomy catheter is inserted to keep the track open. After repeated X-ray examination for control, more stones can be looked for at another time.

Percutaneous kidney stone surgery, in terms of its principles, its anatomico surgical conditions, and its risks, puts everything that has been taken for granted in kidney surgery in a new light.

B. Topography of the Percutaneous Track

The percutaneous approach to the kidney runs through the retroperitoneal space. The direction of the puncture corresponds to the lateral position of the kidney, running a slightly lateral-dorsal to medial-ventral course. This approach ensures that the puncture needle reaches the kidney and the collecting system without injuring the large vessels at the hilus. Fluoroscopy would otherwise show that the needle had gone right through the entire kidney. For the approach via the lower pole of the kidney, which is the most commonly used access, only the muscles are penetrated, apart from the skin and subcutaneous fatty tissue, before the perinephrium and the kidney are reached. This track is situated caudal to the middle of the kidney and thus below the tip of the 12th rib. This nearly rules out the danger of puncturing the pleural cavity. Should a calyx from the middle group have to be punctured for topographic reasons, however, the pleura could be injured, since the intercostal space 11–12 often has to be used for the puncture. This can happen rather easily when

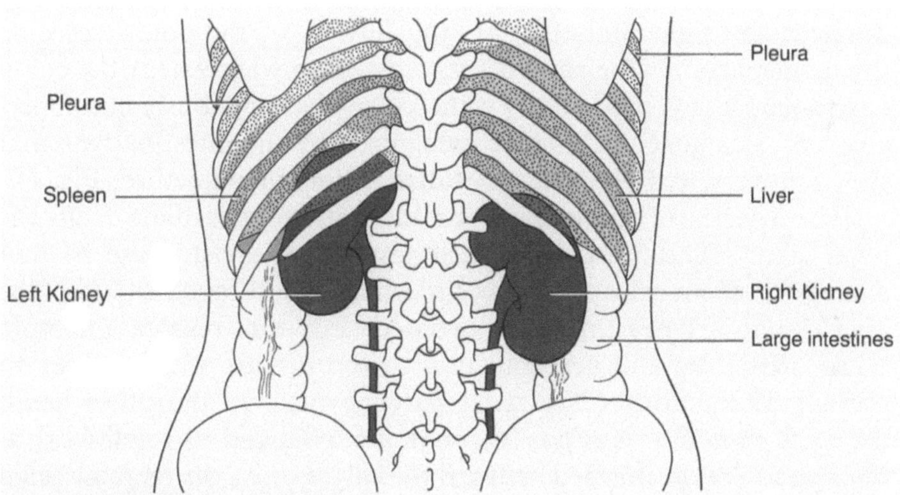

Fig. 1. Topography of the kidney

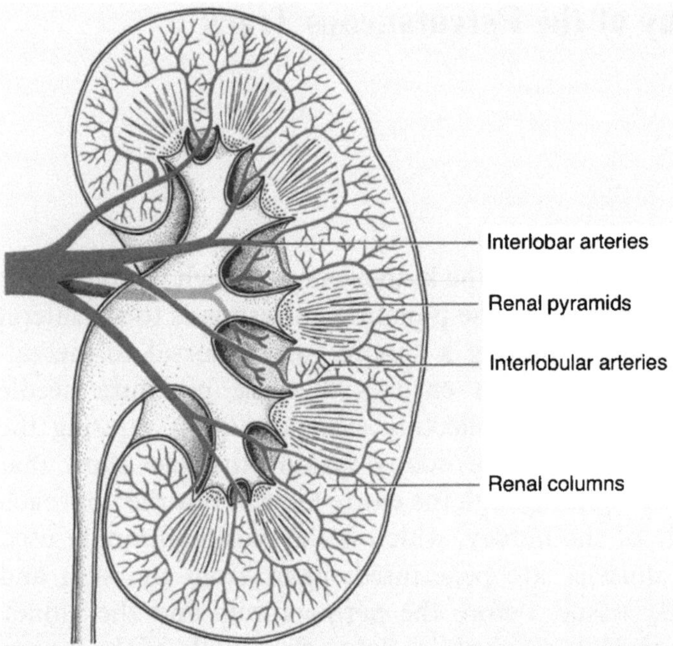

Fig. 2. Arterial vascular supply of the kidney in ventral view. Only few arterial vessels are affected when the percutaneous track through a papilla is laid perpendicular to the surface of the kidney

the left side is being punctured, as the left kidney is higher than the right and its uppermost pole is crossed by the 11th rib. Ventrally on both the right and the left, the flexura of the colon rests on the perinephrium. One should try to assess to what extent the colon covers the kidney, particularly if the kidney has previously been operated on. This generally can be recognized by the intestinal gas that shows up very well on the X-ray taken during the puncture (Fig. 1).

The arteries of the kidney, for the most part, radiate from the renal artery. The 5 segmental arteries do not anastomose so that damage to them, also at the point where they branch off into the interlobular arteries, must be avoided. For this reason, puncture tracks should be laid perpendicular to the surface of the kidney to prevent destruction of the renal parenchyma. On the other hand, the track should always pass through a papilla and its related calyx, since punctures performed between the calyces, i.e., between the renal columns, cause damage to the arteries located in that area (Fig. 2).

C. Position and Preparation of the Patient

The patient is positioned on a urological X-ray table equipped with an image amplifier. This enables the surgeon to control the position of the stone and the pyeloscope on the monitor at any time during the operation. The image, however, is only in one plane, as the tube is usually not moveable. The patient is always positioned on his stomach with the body kept straight and flat on both sides. This keeps the track from kinking and the nephrostomy catheter from sliding out of the kidney when the patient is repositioned later on. A pillow placed under the side of an obese patient may not effect any change at all, but the same pillow under a thin person could raise the side of the body by 45°. The surgeon has to know that all patients, regardless of their figures, are in the same position, especially if the surgical sheets make it impossible to see the exact position. In this way, the surgeon can get used to working with the same topographic conditions and can spot any deviation in the direction of the track.

With very obese patients, there is the chance that the pyeloscope will not be long enough to reach the kidney. In this case, a thick pillow can be placed under the chest and the pelvis, which will allow the belly to sag. Under these conditions, it will almost always be possible to achieve a percutaneous lithotripsy using a normal pyeloscope.

There should always be a catheter in the bladder during percutaneous operations, as the pressure of the irrigant can cause the bladder to fill rapidly. Despite continuous suction of the irrigant throughout the operation, the flow of large amounts of water cannot be avoided, particularly if the instrument is frequently withdrawn from the percutaneous track or if the lens is removed from the sheath. The fluid sometimes flows over the patient's skin and the surgical sheets. It is therefore essential that the X-ray table be water-proofed. This also applies particularly to the image amplifying tube and the camera, should there be one. Water-proof covers alone cannot adequately protect these sensitive instruments.

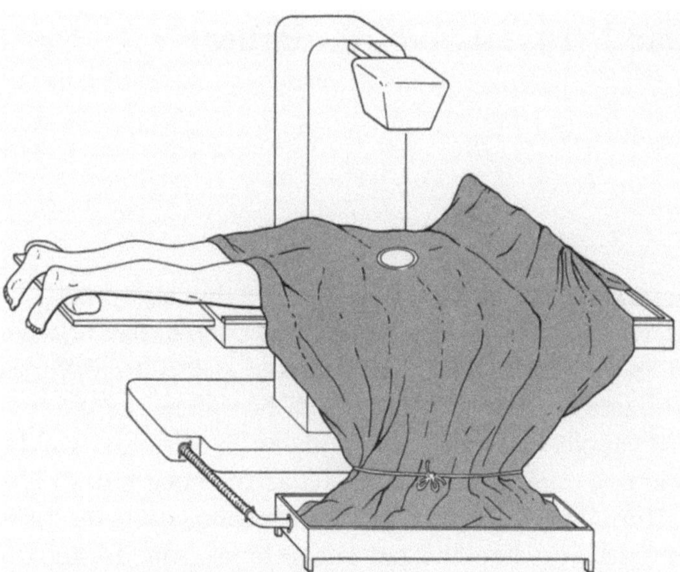

Fig. 3. The patient is positioned on the stomach. The surgical drapes are tied together and hang into a basin where excess water is collected

If there is no drain in the floor of the operating room, the entire floor will be covered with water at the end of the operation. We recommend the following to overcome this problem: a large basin is placed under the table on the side being operated on. If possible, the basin should be connected to the gully of the table with an easy to release bayonet joint. The surgical sheets should be just long enough so that they can hang in the basin when tied together. This way any excess water can flow directly into the basin. We have found this procedure to be quite effective (Fig. 3).

D. Anesthesia

We perform all of our percutaneous operations under local anesthesia. Since most patients find lying on their stomach unpleasant, good sedation with a neuroleptic or a tranquilizer is important. Depending on how long the operation lasts, the sedatives have to be readministered. The area from the skin up to the surface of the kidney is anesthetized with 40 ml of 0.5% lidocain solution. Particular care must be taken that the lumbodorsal fascia is well anesthetized. Young people, who still have firm fasciae, find it unpleasant when the dilators penetrate these fasciae. Dilatation from an intercostal approach can be very painful because the ribs are so close. This can be alleviated by a routine incision made with the guided double blade knife, which considerably facilitates dilation of the track. Entry into the kidney itself is only painful in case of an acute pyelonephritic kidney, as a result of dilatation, for example.

If the track from a previous operation is being used, the renal cavity can be sufficiently anesthetized by the percutaneous administration of lidocain gel (Instillagel, Farco-Pharma), in addition to the local anesthesia. The anesthesia thereby achieved is comparable to that used for the urethra. Even electrohydraulic stone disintegration is tolerable. Should the pyeloscope have to be twisted during the operation, there is going to be some amount of pain, even under a good anesthetic. This requires repeated injections of the sedatives.

E. X-Ray Protection

The patient's pelvic area is covered with a lead apron (on the side towards the X-ray tube!). The surgeon and all personnel wear the usual X-ray aprons. It is advisable for the surgeon to wear lead glass goggles, at least while laying the percutaneous track. Special hand protection is still not available.

It is of utmost importance that as little as possible be X-rayed. Furthermore, the X-ray field should be focussed so precisely that only the actual operation is visible. The danger of radiation exposure must be taken seriously, as a difficult operation can mean more than 30 min screening time. A special safety device is presently being prepared which will provide a protective wall between the X-rayed area and the X-ray tube as well as between the operating area and the surgeon. The rigid wall can be sterilized and can be adjusted according to the patient's body. Radiation exposure will thus be reduced to a minimum.

F. Pyeloscope and Further Percutaneous Instruments

The main problem with percutaneous pyeloscopy is the friability of the mucosa, which bleeds at the slightest touch with a rigid instrument. To keep the blood from obstructing vision, it is essential to have a strong irrigation flow to rinse it away. This, however, can cause pyelorenal reflux, especially in the case of pyelonephritis (Figs. 4, 5). Pyeloscopes have thus been designed that ensure low pressure conditions by controlled permanent suction of the rinsing fluid, which is directed onto the image field. This principle, which has been known in bladder surgery for years as "continuous flow resectoscopes", consists of rinsing through the inner sheath and suction through the outer sheath of a double sheath instrument.

1. Pyeloscope

The pyeloscopes designed by Olympus, Winter & Ibe, Storz and Wolf have fulfilled the essential requirements for the instruments (Figs. 6–10). Complications can occur only if a model is used in which a portion of the irrigant is drawn through the inner sheath under the lens. Heavy bleeding will cause the view to become cloudy due to turbulences.

All 3 companies offer lenses with an angled eyepiece, which permit rigid auxiliary devices such as ultrasound probes, forceps, or additional rigid lenses to be inserted through the track (Figs. 11, 12, 13a, b). For surgery on difficult calyceal calculi or on calculi in the upper ureter, it is absolutely necessary to use an adaptable flexible fiberscope, which can be flexed up to 160°, thus producing an almost retrospect effect should have a sufficient instrumental channel of approximately 5–6 Fr. The instrument and it should also be as thin as possible so that it can pass through the fine structures in the kidney. The sharp flexion of the tip, however, is only possible to a certain degree, since the auxiliary instruments, depending on their quality, can cause additional stiffening of the tip. Furthermore, the

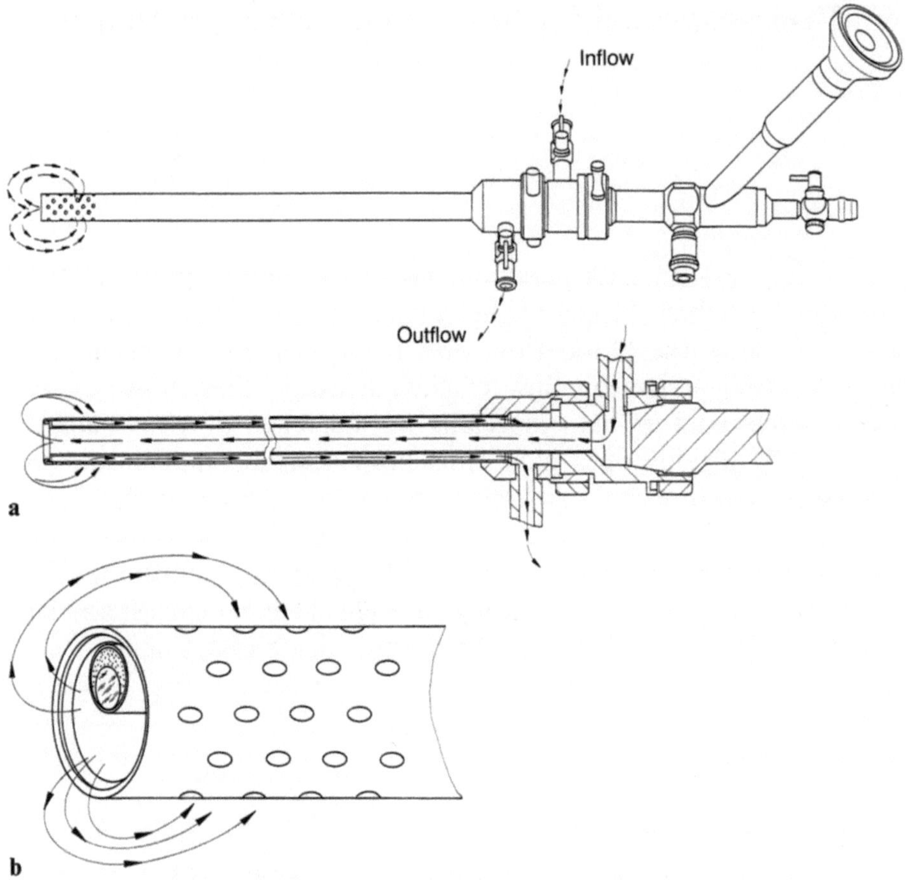

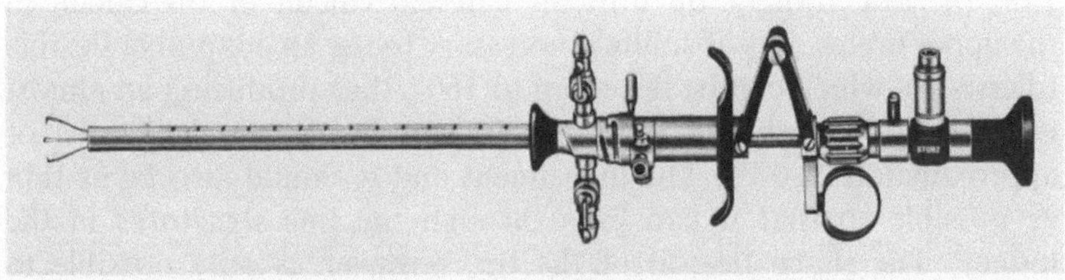

Fig. 4a, b. A double sheath pyeloscope allows good vision, even when there is heavy bleeding. Irrigation takes place through the inner sheath, controlled suction through the outer sheath. Larger stone fragments can also be removed by shifting irrigation to the outer sheath and suction to the instrument channel (Olympus, Winter & Ibe)

Fig. 5. Pyeloscope (Storz) 27 Fr. Size includes grasping forceps developed by Wickham

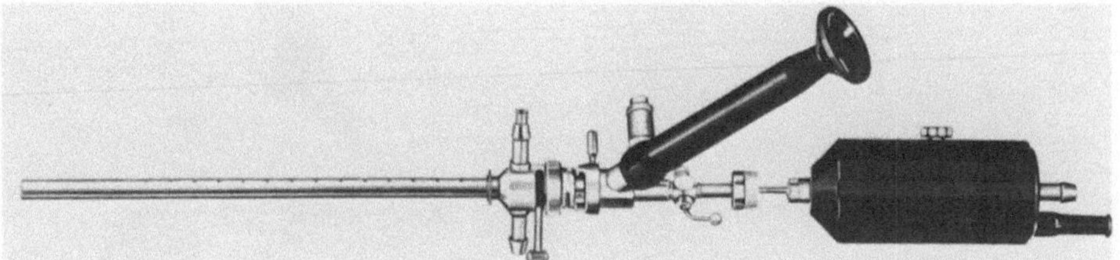

Fig. 6. Pyeloscope (Storz) with angled eyepiece and ultrasound probe inserted

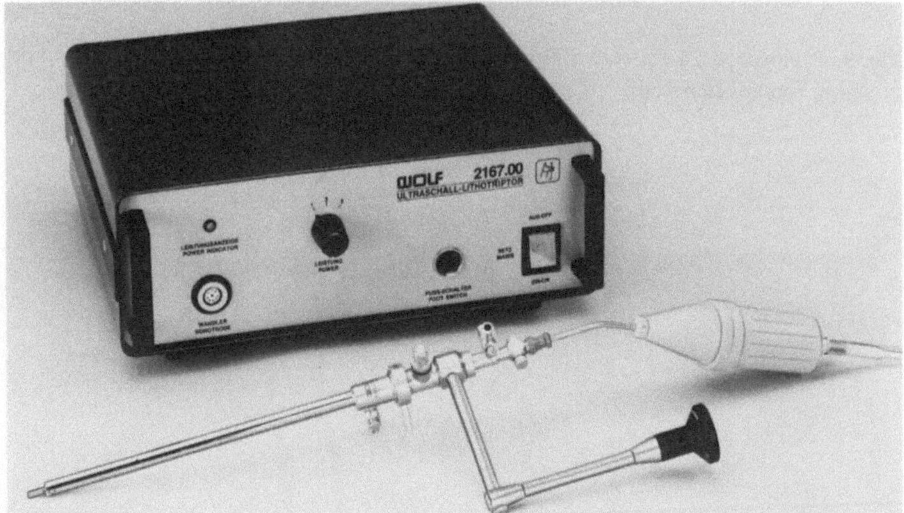

Fig. 7. Pyeloscope (Wolf) with double right-angled eyepiece and ultrasound probe inserted

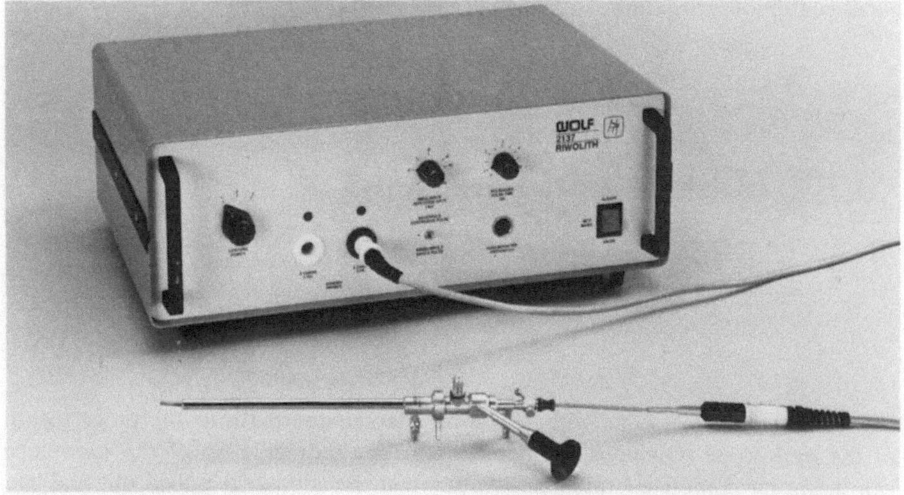

Fig. 8. Pyeloscope (Wolf) with eyepiece at 45° angle and ultrasound probe inserted

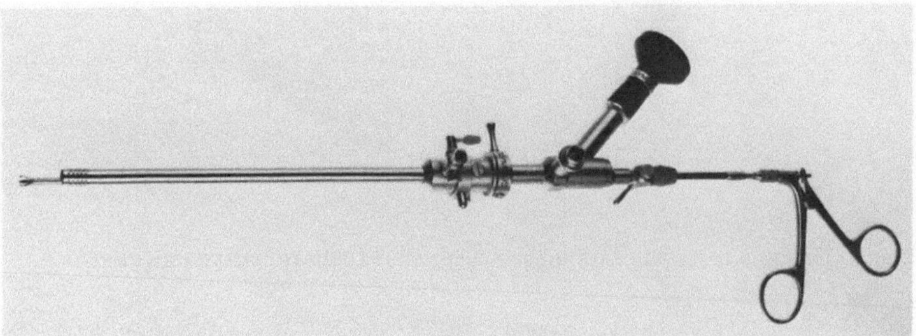

Fig. 9. Pyeloscope 24 Fr. (Olympus, Winter & Ibe) with eyepiece angled at 45° and grasping forceps inserted

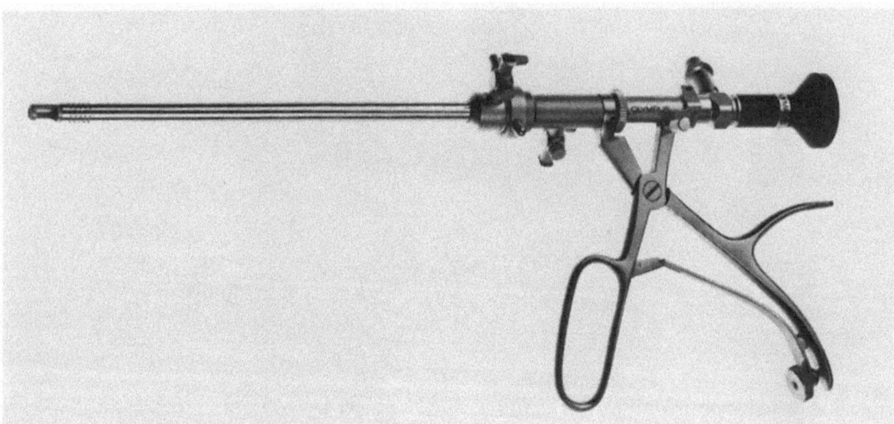

Fig. 10. Pyeloscope (Olympus, Winter & Ibe) with stone punch inserted. Also provides continuous irrigation

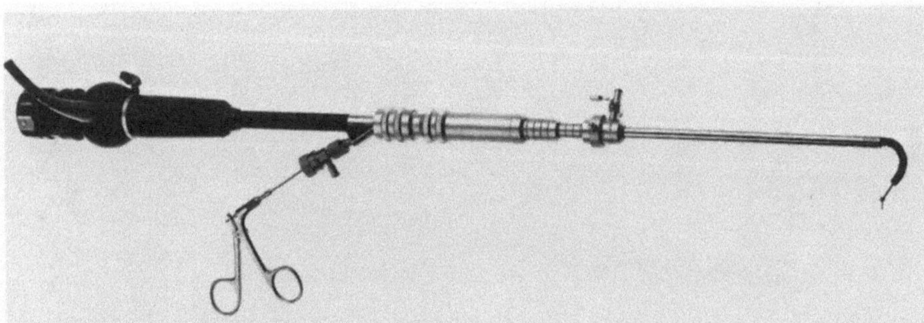

Fig. 11. Flexible fiberscope with telescope adapter inserted into the outer sheath of the pyeloscope (Olympus, Winter & Ibe). The moveable tip of the endoscope can disappear completely into the sheath when the adapter is pulled out and can be advanced 7 cm when the adapter is pushed in

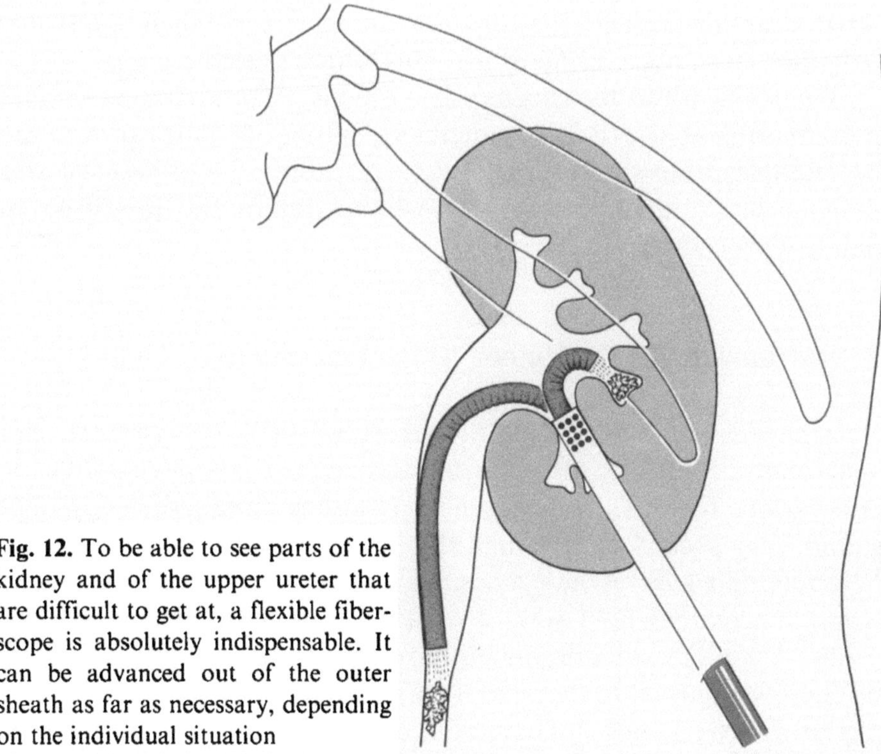

Fig. 12. To be able to see parts of the kidney and of the upper ureter that are difficult to get at, a flexible fiberscope is absolutely indispensable. It can be advanced out of the outer sheath as far as necessary, depending on the individual situation

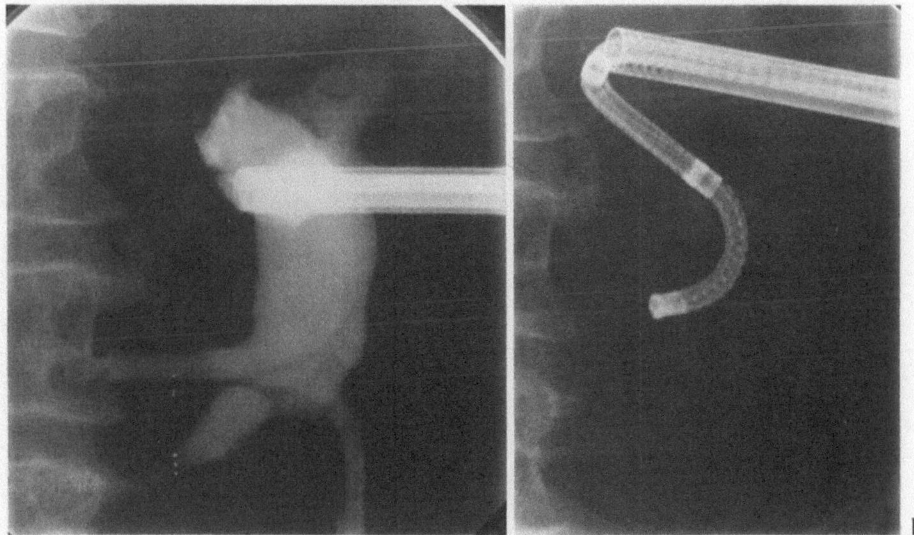

Fig. 13a, b. Inspection of the cavity system of a horseshoe kidney after stone removal. The tip of the flexible fiberscope is extended its full length of 7 cm corresponding to the course of the cavity system

flexion can obstruct the instrument channel completely and adequate irrigation in the case of bleeding is no longer possible.

Operating a flexible lens requires practice. To learn the technique it is advisable to use the instrument as a matter of routine for urethrocystoscopies, thus on an organ whose anatomy the urologist is very familiar with (and any young man will be grateful for this absolutely painless procedure).

2. Instruments for the Kidney Stone Operation

For the extraction of simple kidney stones it is necessary to have a selection of flexible, soft, Dormia baskets, a stone punch (Fig. 14), and various forceps. Larger stones are either disintegrated by ultrasound, then sucked out through the probe, or one can apply electrohydraulic shockwaves via probes, which are available in sizes ranging from approximately 4.5 Fr. to 10 Fr. The thin electrohydraulic probes are more suitable for employment in the flexible fiberscope because, in contrast to the rigid ultrasound probe, they make it possible to destroy stones that are difficult to get at and still provide a sufficient cleansing stream.

Ultrasound instruments are available from Wolf and Storz. Electrohydraulic devices are manufactured by Wolf, (Figs. 15 and 16) Northgate (Distributor ACMI), Walz and Urat. Urat has come out with a new combination device (Baikal) for electrohydraulic shockwaves and ultrasonic waves which has a flexible probe. However, to date there have been no reports on experiences with this instrument.

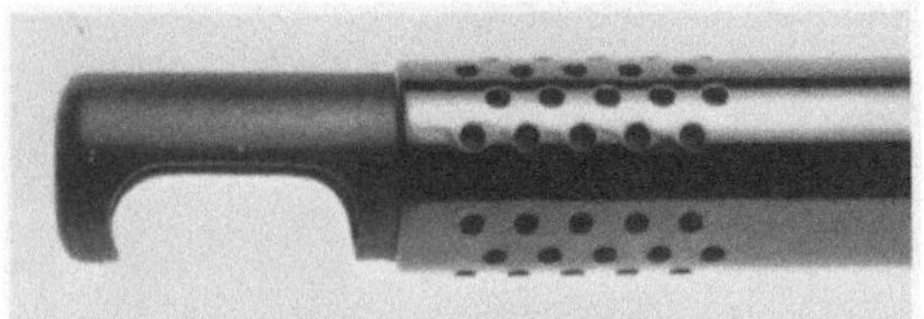

Fig. 14. The stone punch is ideal for the mechanical disintegration of relatively small pelvic stones

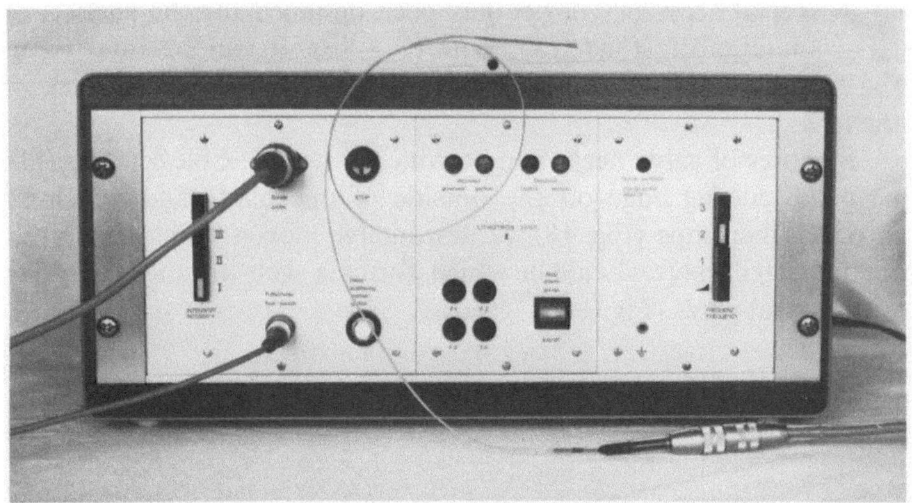

Fig. 15. The electrohydraulic device from Walz (Lithotron 2000)

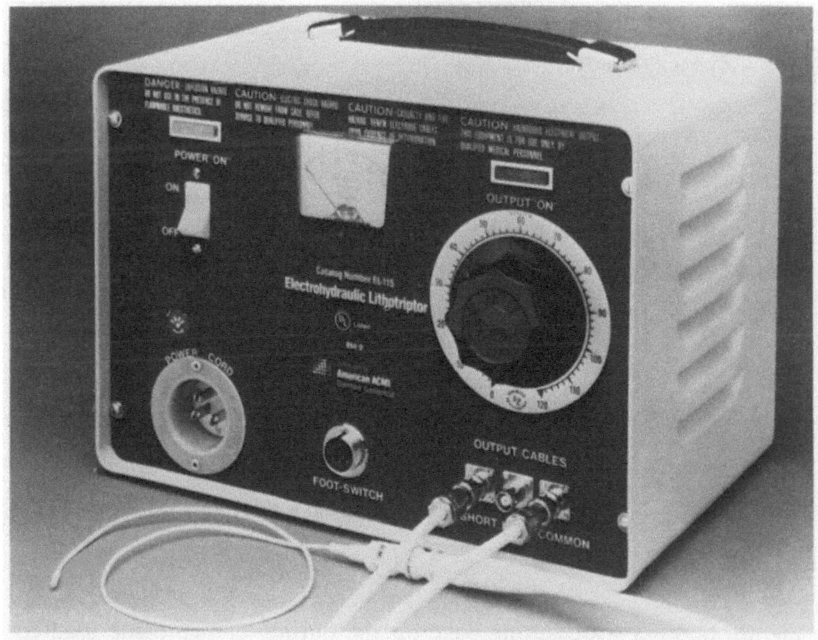

Fig. 16. Electrohydraulic stone disintegrator from Northgate (distributed by ACMI)

A special accessory device has been designed for the suction of large amounts of stone fragments (Fig. 17). It can be inserted in the sheath of the Olympus, Winter & Ibe pyeloscope in place of the lens.

Stenoses of calyx necks can be widened with flexible scissors that have the cutting edge on the outside of one blade and which fit into the fiberscope (Fig. 18). A new, active loop is being developed for impacted calyceal calculi which forms a web around the stone with several wires (Fig. 19).

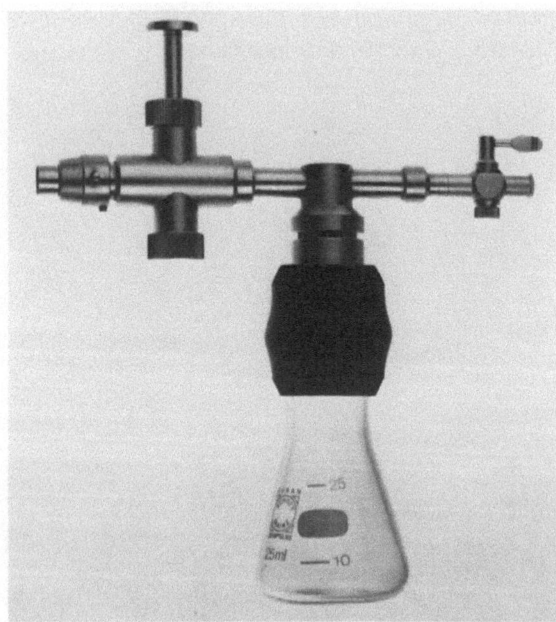

Fig. 17. Large stone fragments can be sucked out through the inner sheath without direct vision if a suction device controlled with a trumpet valve is inserted in place of the lens

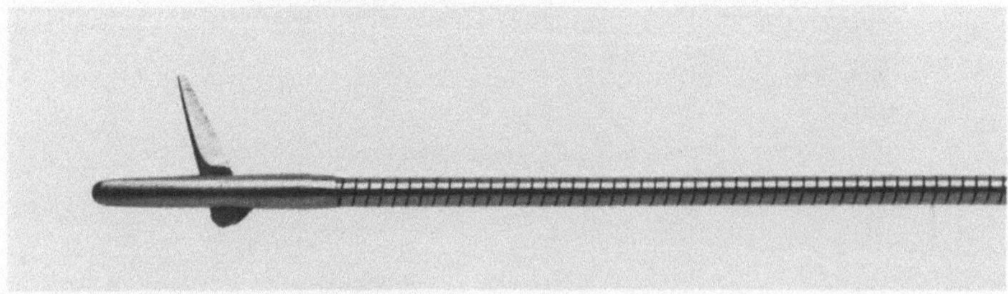

Fig. 18. Scissors with cutting edge on the outside of one blade used for opening narrow calyx necks or for perforating a neighboring calyx

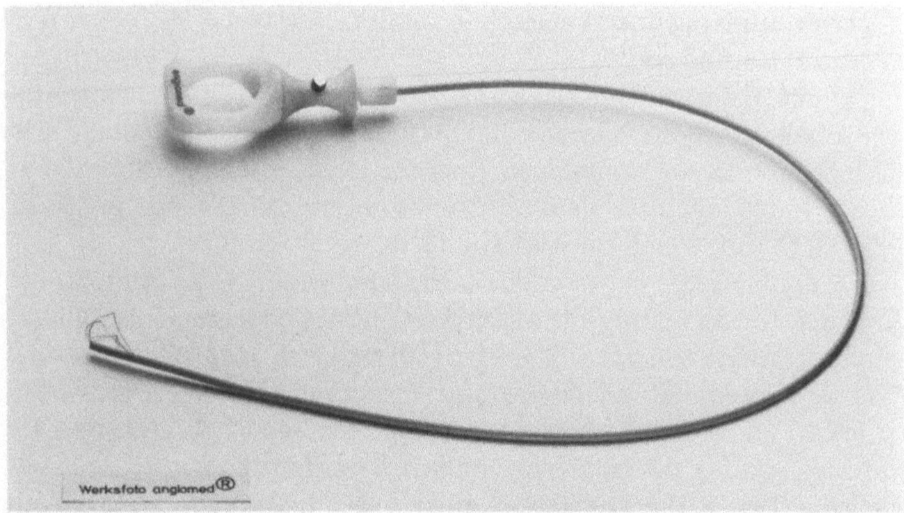

Fig. 19. A new "active loop" is being designed with several wires to surround and grasp the stone and with one single wire for use in calyx necks. The handle can be removed and further advancing of the wire causes it to form a web around the stone. This is done without direct vision

3. Instruments for Percutaneous Puncture and Dilatation

A triple needle developed by Günther (available from Angiomed or Vance) is used for kidney punctures. A Chiba needle is also suitable (Figs. 20 and 21). We use a double needle with a dull outer needle and a sharp inner needle. Flexible guide wires, such as those commonly used in angiography, are advanced through the outer needle (Figs. 22 and 23). These wires – Seldinger or Lunderquist guide wires – have a diameter of 0.35 mm and a J-shaped tip. Seldinger wires adapt well to the anatomic conditions of the kidney, however, since they are soft, they often bend when guiding a dilator through the fasciae and the muscles. The Lunderquist wires are better suited for this purpose, as they are stiff and allow the dilator to pass easily. They have a soft, flexible tip which conforms well to the shape of the kidney. However, they can cause perforation of the calyx.

The percutaneous track can be dilated with teflon dilators (Angiomed or Vance), which are available in sizes up to 28 Fr. (Fig. 24). The disadvantage of these dilators is that the thin ones are very soft and can easily bend when penetrating strong fasciae (Fig. 25).

I prefer applying metal telescope dilators (designed by Alken) via a central leading rod.

If one plans to begin the actual stone operation immediately after the track has been dilated, one should leave a second guide wire parallel to the instrument so that the percutaneous track can be easily found again. This wire can be inserted via a special 24 Fr. dilatation rod, which fits over the 18 Fr. rod (Fig. 25a).

A double knife led by a guide wire and equipped with an adjustable disc for regulating the distance facilitates passage of the dilators along the guide wire (Fig. 26). This is particularly helpful if the kidney has been operated on before and the fascia and muscle tissue is scarred. The knife is used to cut a 10 mm wide slit through the fasciae. Turning the knife while pulling it out produces a cross-shaped incision (Fig. 27). A so-called Amplatz sheath made of polyurethane helps keep the percutaneous track open for the duration of an operation performed in one session.

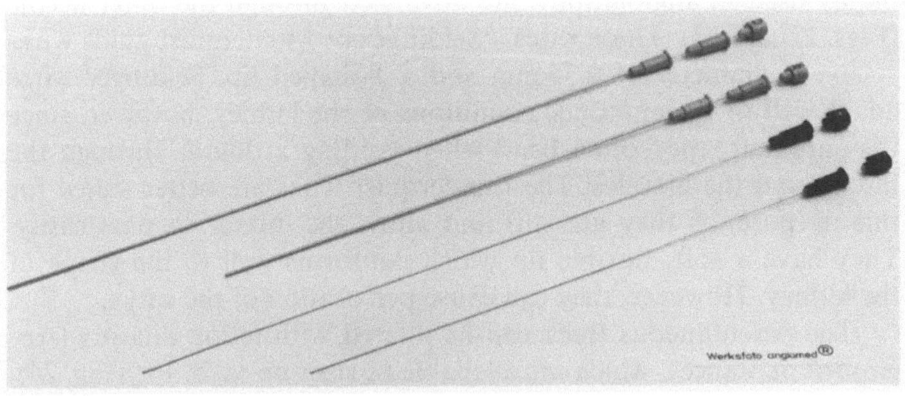

Fig. 20. *Above:* 3-piece puncture needle developed by Günther, outer diameter 1.3 mm. *Below:* 2-piece thin needle by Chiba. Outer diameter 0.7 mm

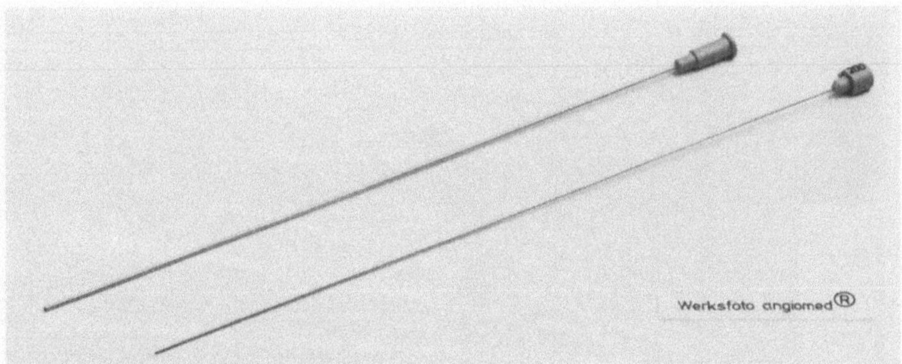

Fig. 21. Two-piece puncture needle, "Loretto" model, with outer diameter of 1.3 mm

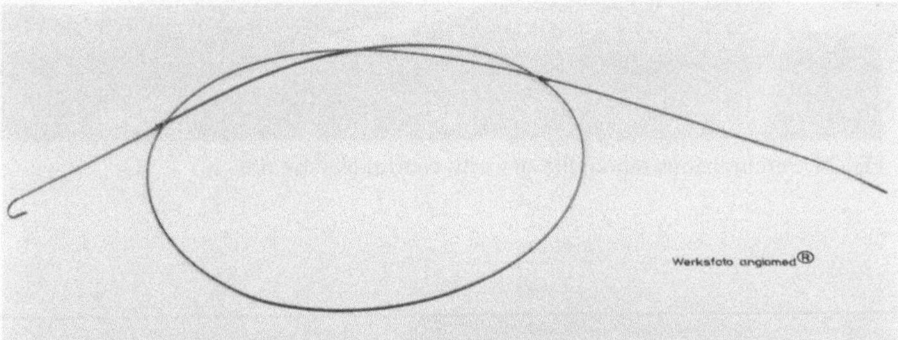

Fig. 22. Seldinger wire with 0.35 mm diameter and J-tip

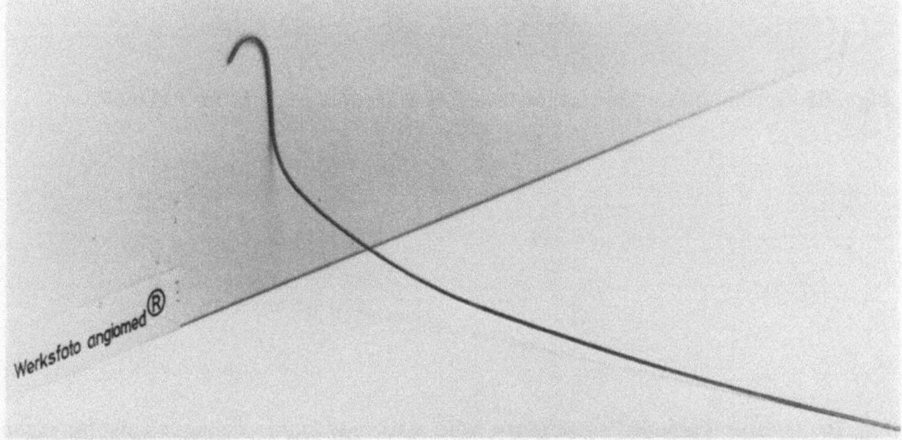

Fig. 23. Lunderquist wire with semi-stiff sheath and soft J-tip; 0.35 mm in diameter

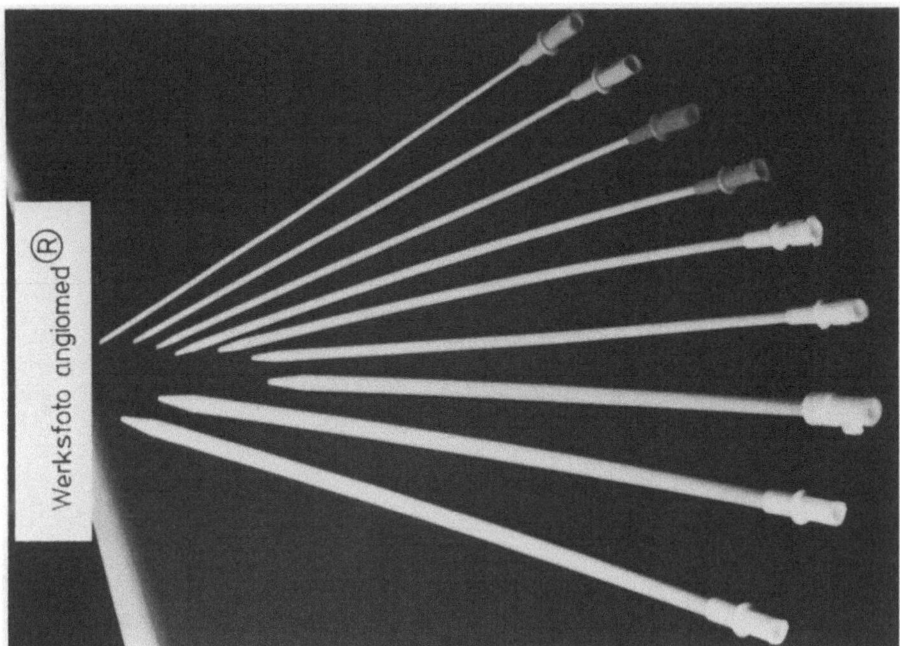

Fig. 24. Percutaneous teflon dilators with central leading rod

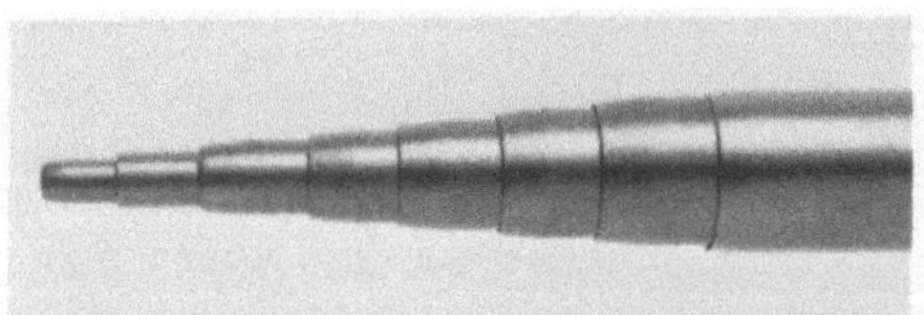

Fig. 25a. Metal dilators of the telescope dilator set with tips on top of one another

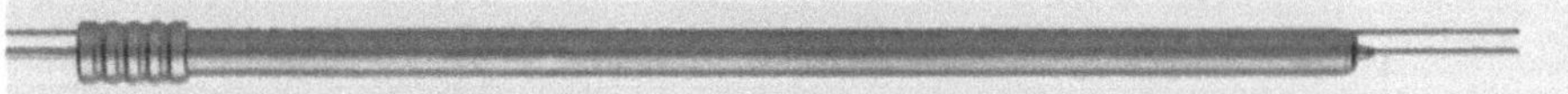

Fig. 25b. Special dilatation rod for inserting a second guide (after LeDuc)

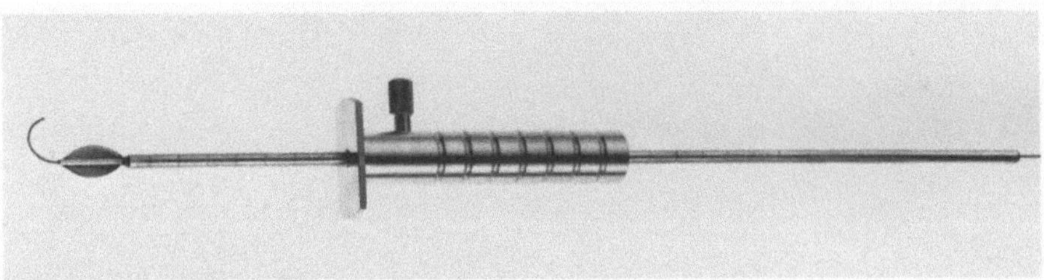

Fig. 26. Double knife led by a guide wire with adjustable distance ring for clean separation of muscle and scar plates

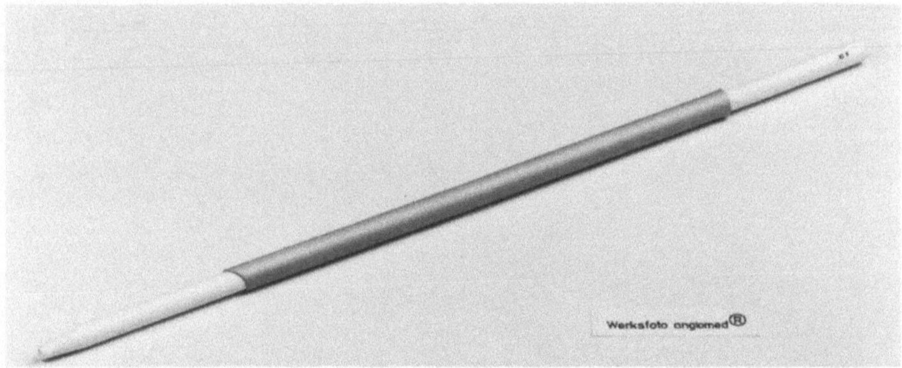

Fig. 27. Amplatz sheath keeps the percutaneous track open during the operation

4. Irrigation and Suction

Physiological saline solutions or electrolyte-free solutions such as Purisole (Sorbitol & Mannitol, Fresenius) or Glycocoll (Travenol) are good irrigants for pyeloscopy. With electrolyte-free solutions, there might be a problem with the spark discharge at the tip when electrohydraulic shockwaves are applied. Northgate recommends the following solutions to be used with its instruments:

1. 6 ml concentrated sodium chloride injection solution (23.4%) per liter of sterile water

   or

2. 1.4 grams sodium chloride (NaCl molecular weight 58.44) per liter of sterile water

   or

3. 0.9% sodium chloride diluted at a ratio of 1:6 with sterile water.

   When the rigid pyeloscope is used, the bag containing the irrigant is hung 40–60 cm above the instrument. With the flexible pyeloscope, the irrigant bag is hung as high as possible to allow minimum irrigation when instruments are inserted into the working channel.

   The irrigant is sucked out of the pyeloscope by means of a normal, controllable pump, such as the kind used for transurethral resection or in the operating room. Adjusting the respective stopcock on the pyeloscope regulates the suction.

G. Puncture of the Kidney

The art of laying a good percutaneous track is probably the most important prerequisite for the success of a percutaneous kidney stone operation. A mislaid track can make it necessary to interrupt the operation to find a better track. A stone in the upper part of the ureter, for example, could hardly be reached if the track led into the kidney via the lower pole. Directing the instrument into the upper ureter requires keeping the angle as flat as possible. Even the flexible fiberscope is of no help here, since experience has shown that calculi in the upper ureter are difficult to move and stronger instruments are needed to get them out. It can also be a problem to remove a calyceal stone in a middle calyx group if a neighboring calyx which covers over the stone and possibly over the entire calyx is erroneously selected for puncture.

It is thus essential that the position of the track be carefully and strategically planned in order to make the operation itself as uncomplicated as possible. If the track is well laid, the operation may only have to consist of getting hold of the stone and extracting it.

1. Puncture of a Dilated Kidney

A dilated kidney can usually be punctured with no difficulty under the guidance of an ultrasound device (Fig. 28). The cavity system is filled with urine and the ultrasound image gives an adequate demonstration of a suitable calyx. X-ray control is only necessary for dilatation.

2. Puncture of a Nondilated Kidney

If the cavity system is not dilated, the walls of the calyces lie against one another, making it difficult to insert a needle in between them, particularly under ultrasound control alone. It is advisable in this

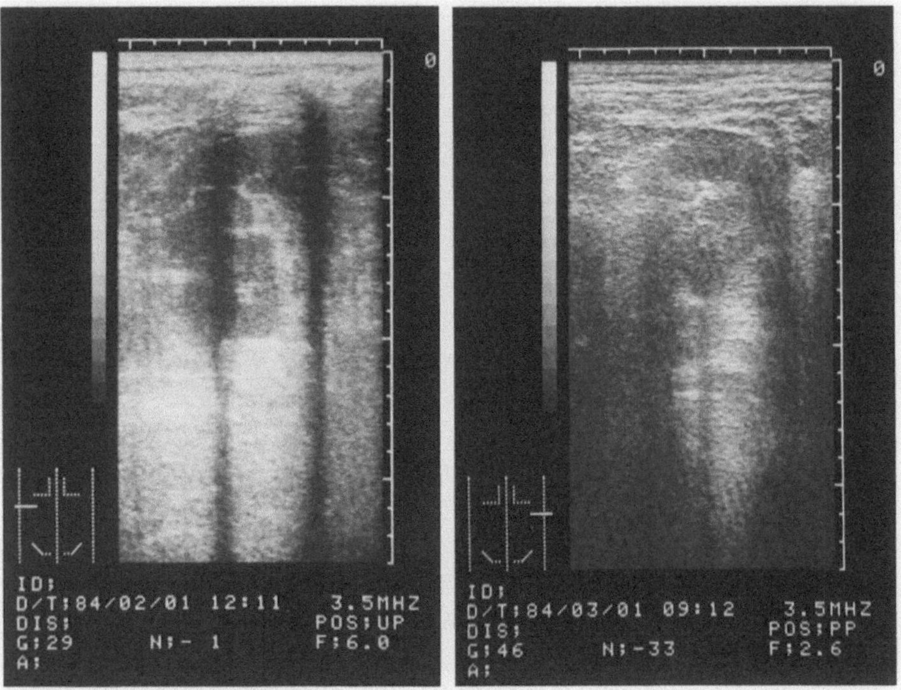

Fig. 28   **Fig. 29**

Fig. 28. A dilated kidney can be punctured with no difficulty under ultrasound guidance alone

Fig. 29. Laying the ultrasound probe across the first plane produces the second plane and the point on the skin opposite to the highest point of convexity of the kidney. This point is usually on the posterior axillary line. In this case a dilated calyx can be seen intercostally, under-neath the reflection of the stone, and behind it the sound-shadow. In such a case the right calyx can be punctured under ultrasound guidance alone

case to use the following procedure: a normal 5 Fr. ureteral catheter is inserted retrograde into the renal pelvis and a mixture of 30% contrast agent and 1 or 2 ampoules of indigo carmine is infused into the renal cavity system. This results in a slight hydronephrotic expansion of the cavity system and a strong coloring of the actual puncture target by the contrast. The individual calyces can be hit more easily and more exactly. As soon as the tip of the needle has reached the inside of a calyx, blue dye drips out of the needle. The position of the tip of the needle is then certain and one avoids a possible parapelvine injection of contrast agent, which could obscure the image of the kidney on the X-ray.

Puncture of the kidney is carried out on the urological X-ray table described above and thus in one plane (Fig. 29). The second plane is produced by laying the ultrasound probe across the first plane. The most favorable point for the position of the percutaneous track is indicated by the highest point of convexity. A too tangential approach must be avoided, since it could result in serious vessel damage, particularly if puncture and dilatation have veered off too far ventral. When the ultrasound probe contains a central puncture track, the calyx that harbors the stone can be repeatedly demonstrated and punctured.

Usually, however, the ideal approach to the calyx in question is never found by ultrasound guidance. It is therefore better to carry out the actual puncture under X-ray control. If the needle is positioned correctly in the PA ray path but too far ventral in the other plane, one can detect this by moving the tip of the needle and observing how the large intestine moves (Fig. 30). This can be recognized by the shaking motion of the intestinal gas. The needle is pulled back a bit and advanced towards the kidney in the dorsal direction. Generally, the kidney is then reached right away. The rapid motion of the tip of the needle shows that the kidney is moving in the same rhythm (Fig. 31). The needle is then gradually advanced to the desired papilla of the calyx, which becomes visibly dented when hit (Fig. 32).

After the needle is advanced further and the mandrin removed, blue dye drips out of the needle. Blood flowing out of the needle usually means that a vein has been punctured. Injected contrast agent can be seen on the X-ray draining medially through the veins. In no case should such a track be dilated. The needle is removed and puncture is started again in order to find a better track (Fig. 33–35).

If the retrograde probing of the renal cavity system is unsuccessful, demonstration has to be carried out in the usual way using an intravenously infused contrast agent. In comparison, however, this demonstration is weak and puncturing a calyx is far more difficult than with retrograde expansion.

The retrograde infusion of contrast into a kidney that is pyelonephritically altered can cause slight pain. This is sometimes the result of a pyelorenal reflux. A diuretic should therefore be administered to strengthen the orthograde flow of urine. The retrograde infusion of contrast and the dilatation of the kidney are generally more successful when a spasmolysant is intravenously administered beforehand.

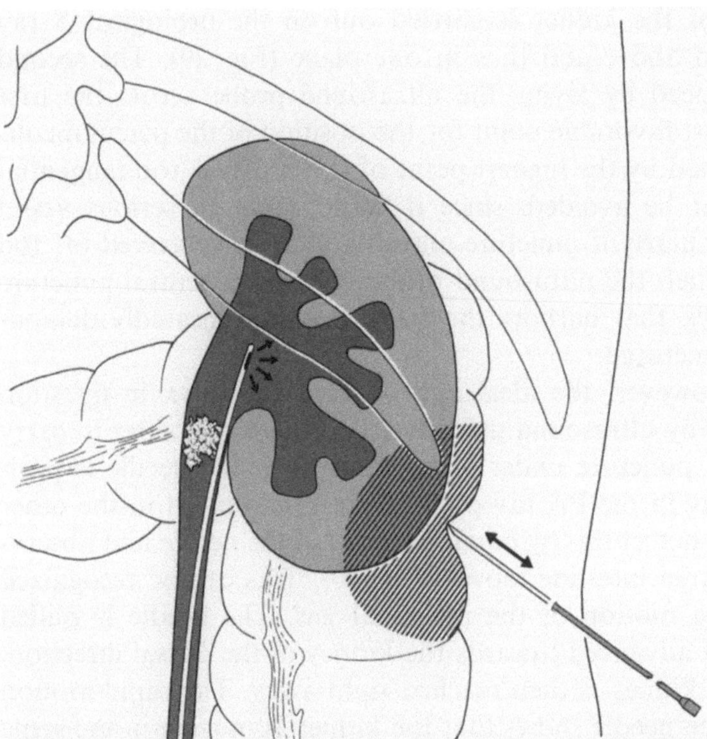

Fig. 30. Puncture of a nondilated renal cavity system. A ureteral catheter is pushed retrograde past the stone and a mixture of 30% contrast agent with indigo carmine is infused into the cavity system, making the target easily recognizable. Blue dye drips out of the needle when the target has been reached. If the tip of the needle is too far ventral from the kidney, the intestine will move in the same rhythm as the needle

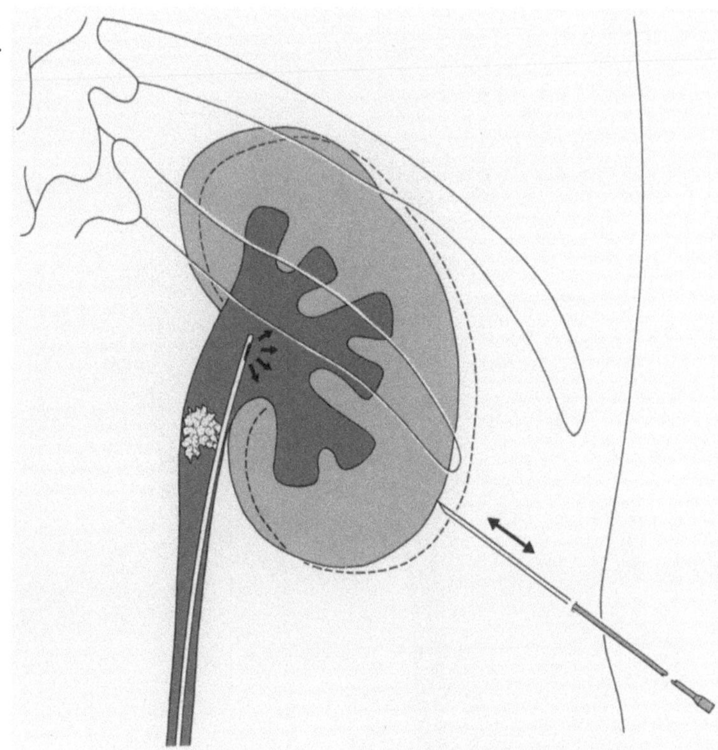

Fig. 31. If the tip of the needle has hit the edge of the kidney, the kidney moves synchronously with the needle

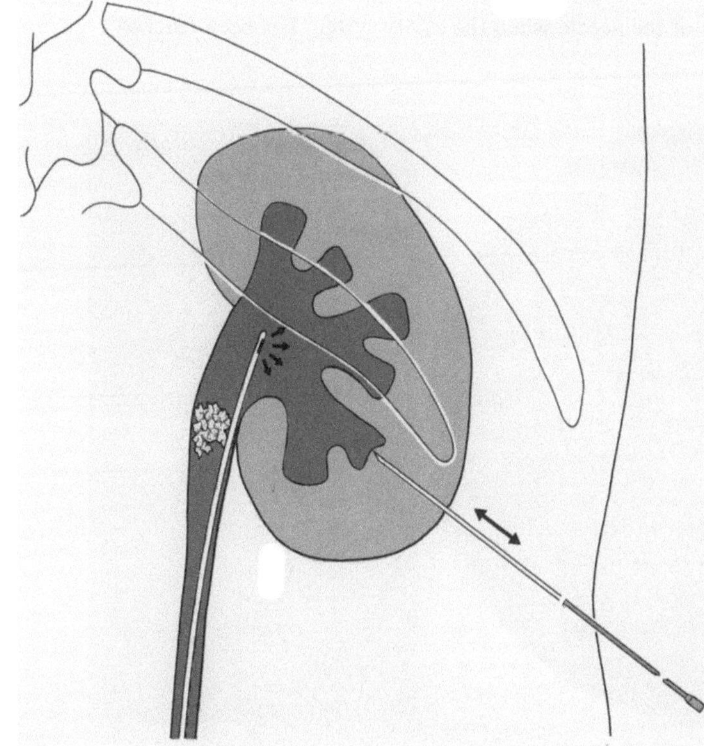

Fig. 32. When the tip of the needle is in the right plane of the desired papilla, slowly advancing the needle will dent the papilla

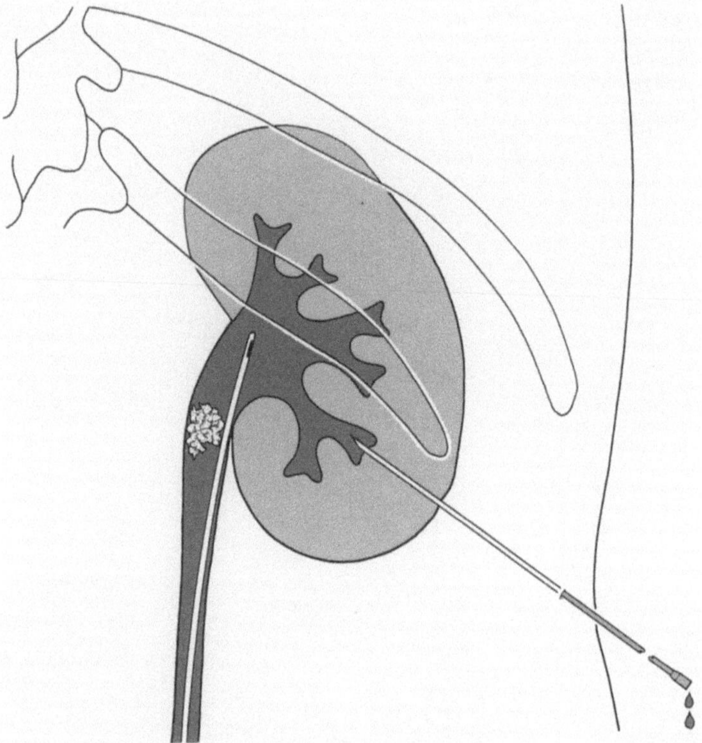

Fig. 33. Blue dye drips out of the needle when the cavity system has been reached

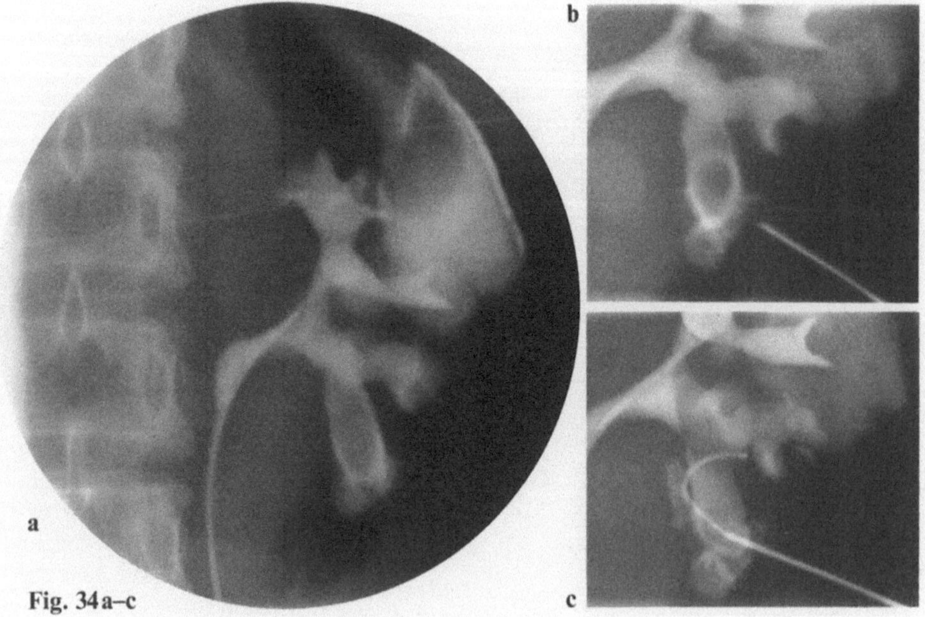

Fig. 34a–c

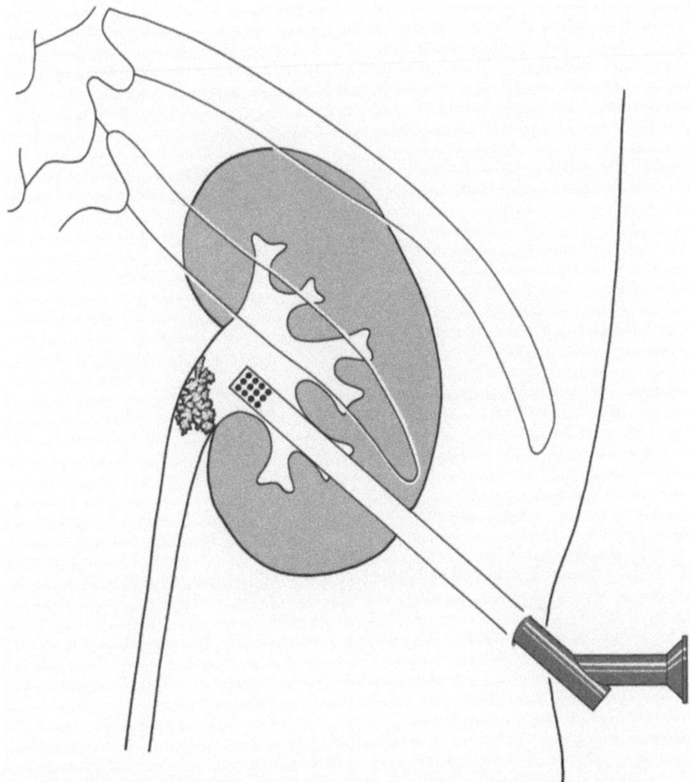

Fig. 35. If the stone operation is to be begun immediately, the outer sheath of the pyeloscope is used in place of the thickest dilation rod

◁ **Fig. 34. a** The cavity system is slightly dilated. Advancing the ureteral catheter too far has caused the tip to go through the calyx and into the renal capsule. **b** The tip of the needle is in the correct position and the papilla is dented when the needle is advanced gradually. **c** Advancing the guide wire

H. Selection of the Percutaneous Track

1. Solitary Pelvic Stones

An approach via a lower calyx neck is usually selected to reach a solitary pelvic stone. If the stone is removed after having been disintegrated rather than in one piece, any existing stone fragments will collect in the lower calyx. They hence lie directly in the track and can easily be extracted. This approach is also the safest, as it is always outside the range of the kidney's contact with the pleura, spleen, and liver.

2. Stone in the Upper Ureter

A percutaneous track that runs through the lower calyx group is not suited for the removal of a stone in the upper ureter, since the pyeloscope would have to be inserted into the ureter at a very sharp angle. Although the rigid pyeloscope can be twisted about 30° in the kidney without difficulty and without damaging the organ, it is usually impossible to drive the instrument into the upper ureter, even when the ureter is dilated. For this reason, an approach via the middle calyx group must be chosen. The calyces on the left side of the group sometimes lie within the lowermost pleura recess. It is therefore necessary to check the X-ray or ultrasonically as to whether there is any danger in laying the track in this area. If so, it is wise to raise the top end of the operating table so that the kidney is dropped. The approach to the middle calyx group is generally made through the lowermost intercostal space (ICS 11–12).

3. Pelvic Stones and Calyceal Stones

To remove a pelvic stone or a calyceal stone in the lower pole region, entry of the percutaneous track must be via the respective calyx.

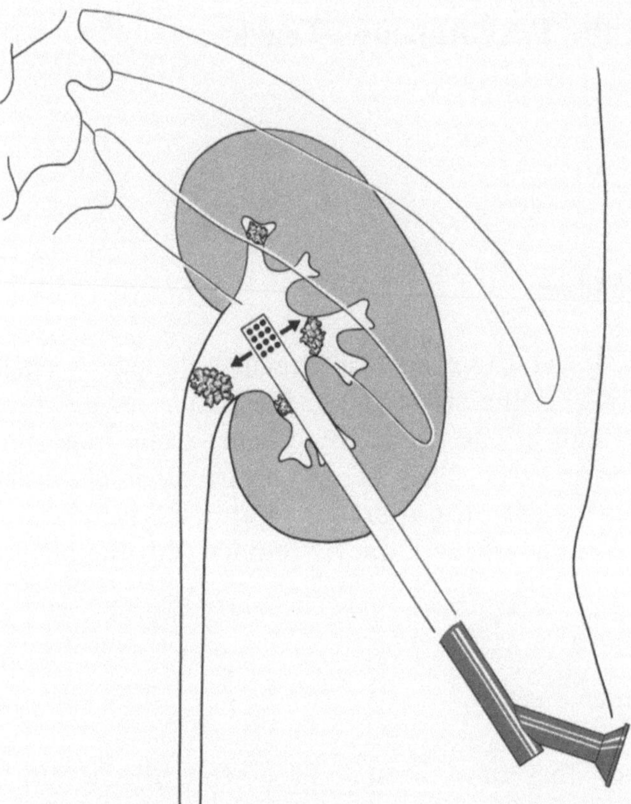

Fig. 36. If possible, all of the stones in the cavity system should be reachable from one percutaneous track. In this case all, the stones are removed by twisting and moving the rigid pyeloscope

The calyceal stone is extracted first and the pyeloscope is then advanced to the pelvic stone. If the calyceal stone is in a calyx of the upper group, the track also has to pass through the lower calyx group so that it runs as straight as possible up to the upper group (Fig. 36).

4. Multiple Calyceal Stones

In selecting the track for multiple calyceal stones, one must try to line up as many of the stones as possible on the one track. Most of the stones can be removed from this track by a slight twisting of the rigid pyeloscope and by applying the flexible fiberscope (Fig. 37).

Fig. 37. Cystine stones in the upper and lower poles of the kidney. Laying the track in the lower calyx group. Tilting the kidney around the sagittal axis made it possible to reach to upper calyx group with the rigid pyeloscope

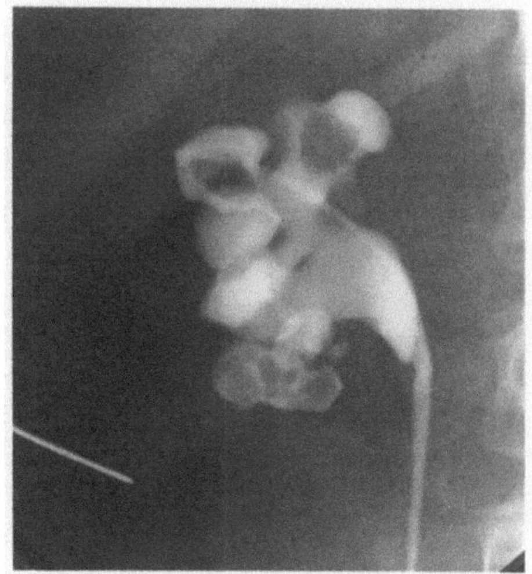

5. Staghorn Stones

In the case of a staghorn stone, a track should be selected through which as much of the stone material as possible can be extracted. If there are stones located in several isolated calyces, 1 or 2 more tracks usually have to be laid. In some cases a neighboring calyx has to be perforated with the surgical instrument. For the first track, however, the lower pole is usually selected so that the major portion of the stone can be removed via this route. This track is kept open until the operation has been completed, even if several sessions are necessary, since remaining stone fragments continue to collect.

J. Dilation of the Puncture Track

1. Normal Anatomic Conditions

After the puncture needle has reached the desired calyx, a flexible guide wire (Seldinger) or a semi-stiff guide wire (Lunderquist) is led through the needle and advanced deep into the kidney (Fig. 38). The track is then dilated, which one can facilitate by dividing the muscles all the way to the renal surface with the double blade knife (see Fig. 26). For this purpose, the distance between the skin and the surface of the kidney is measured beforehand with the ultrasound probe and the distance disc is set accordingly. To cut the track even further than the designated 10 mm, which might be necessary when there is hard scar tissue, the double blade is twisted about 90° at a selected depth and is pulled out. Then the central leading rod of the telescope dilator set or, if teflon dilators are used, the thin dilator is advanced. Since dilatation is done in one plane only, a soft Seldinger guide wire can easily kink in the second plane or can even be pulled out of the kidney through the leading rod or through the first dilator. The wire can be pushed back and forth in the central track with short, quick motions. The wire's refusal to be moved anymore indicates that it has kinked, in which case the affected portion of the wire has to be pulled out through the track. This complication alone makes it advisable, when using Seldinger wires, to advance as much wire as possible into the cavity system.

If the kidney is low or the patient is obese, it is sometimes impossible to achieve a straight line for the puncture track from the incision through the lower kidney pole into the renal pelvis. Although the wire can be advanced into the renal pelvis, it kinks according to the anatomic situation. In this case, if the kidney at least moves easily and has not been operated on before, a tilt around the sagittal axis can be achieved if one inserts the central leading rod through the track, lifts the lower pole of the kidney with the tip, and advances the rod into the renal pelvis. The rod fixates the kidney like a spit and the track is straightened.

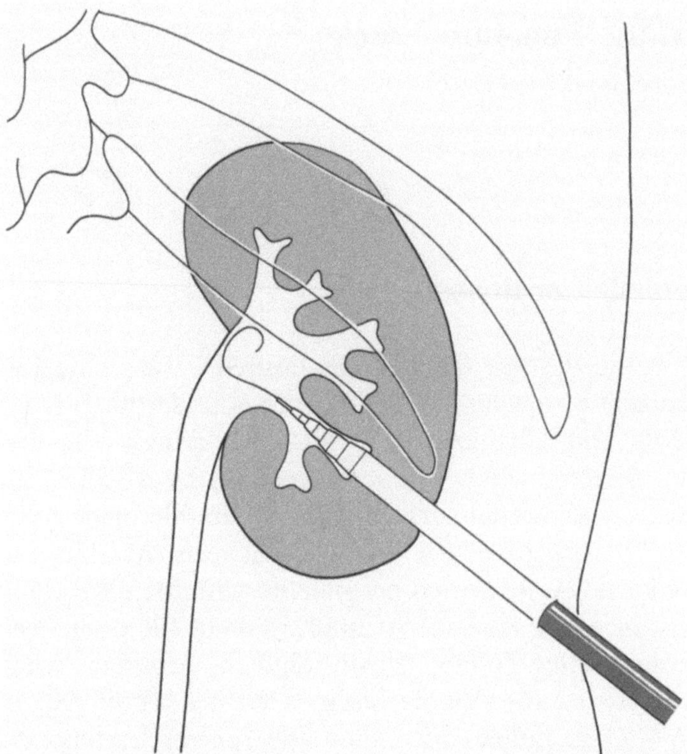

Fig. 38. Inserting the flexible guide wire and dilating the percutaneous track

2. Calyceal Cysts with Small Calyx Necks

When approaching a calculus in a calyceal cyst, it occasionally turns out that the calyx neck is so small that the wire cannot be advanced any further. In this case, the wire should be left in the cyst and the track dilated only up to that point. Forcing the wire may cause perforations of the calyx and loss of the track. This can also result in severe bleeding. After the track has been dilated, the outer sheath of the pyeloscope is inserted instead of the largest dilator. The lens is adjusted and the calyx neck can be found with ease. If the neck is very narrow, it can be cut open immediately with a diathermy knife (in the longitudinal direction of the kidney) and the instrument can be advanced into the renal pelvis. If the neck is not very narrow, the wire under visual control can be passed by the stone, the pyelo-

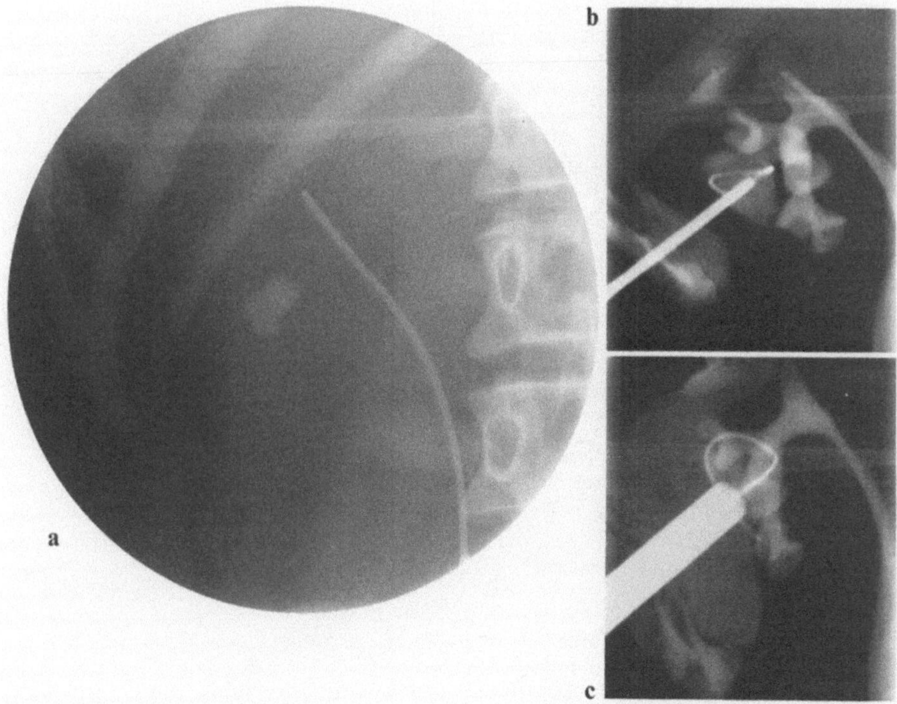

Fig. 39a–c. Puncture of a cystically dilated calyx with stenosis of the calyx neck:
a 2 stones in the lateral calyx **b** Puncture and dilatation **c** Inserting the pyeloscope
(see also color plate I A, B)

scope removed, and dilatation can be continued in the usual manner
(Figs. 39a–c; color plate IA, B).

3. Staghorn Stones and Kidneys with Acute Pyelonephritis

Staghorn stones and acutely infected kidneys should be treated with
antibiotics for 1 to 2 weeks prior to the stone operation. Dilatation
of the track can sometimes lead to an unavoidable lesion of the
mucosa when the nephrostomy catheter is advanced between the
stone and the renal pelvic wall. This brings on chills and fever, just
as in the case of an acutely infected kidney. In this case, it is advisable
to administer a diuretic. Infected renal cavity systems, in particular,
can lead to perforations of the renal pelvis, which results in a via
falsa.

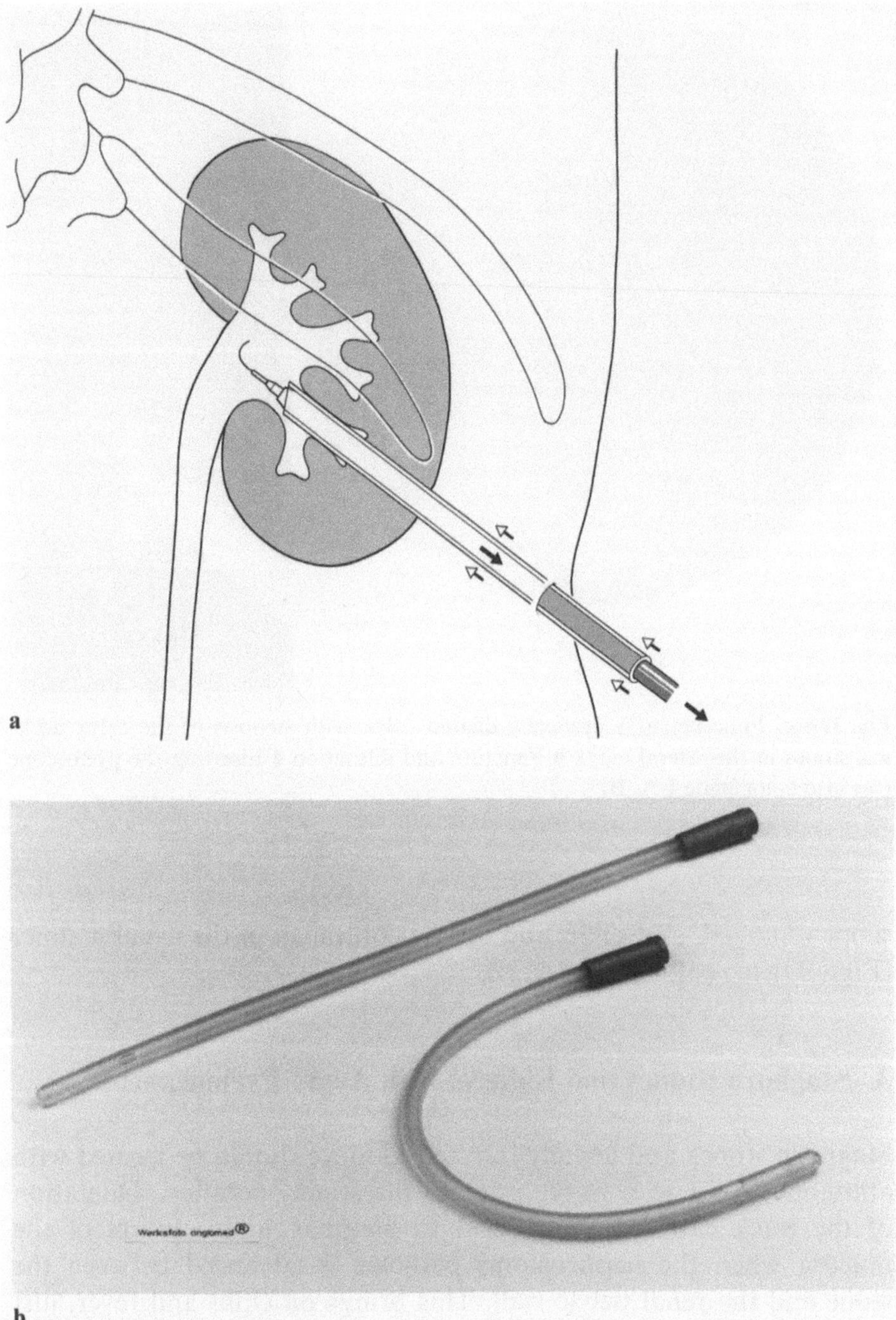

Fig. 40. a After several dilatation rods have been removed, a nephrostomy catheter of the same size is inserted into the track. It is attached to one of the removed dilatation rods so that it becomes stiff and visible on the X-ray. **b** Normal Nelaton catheters made of PVC can be used as nephrostomy catheters

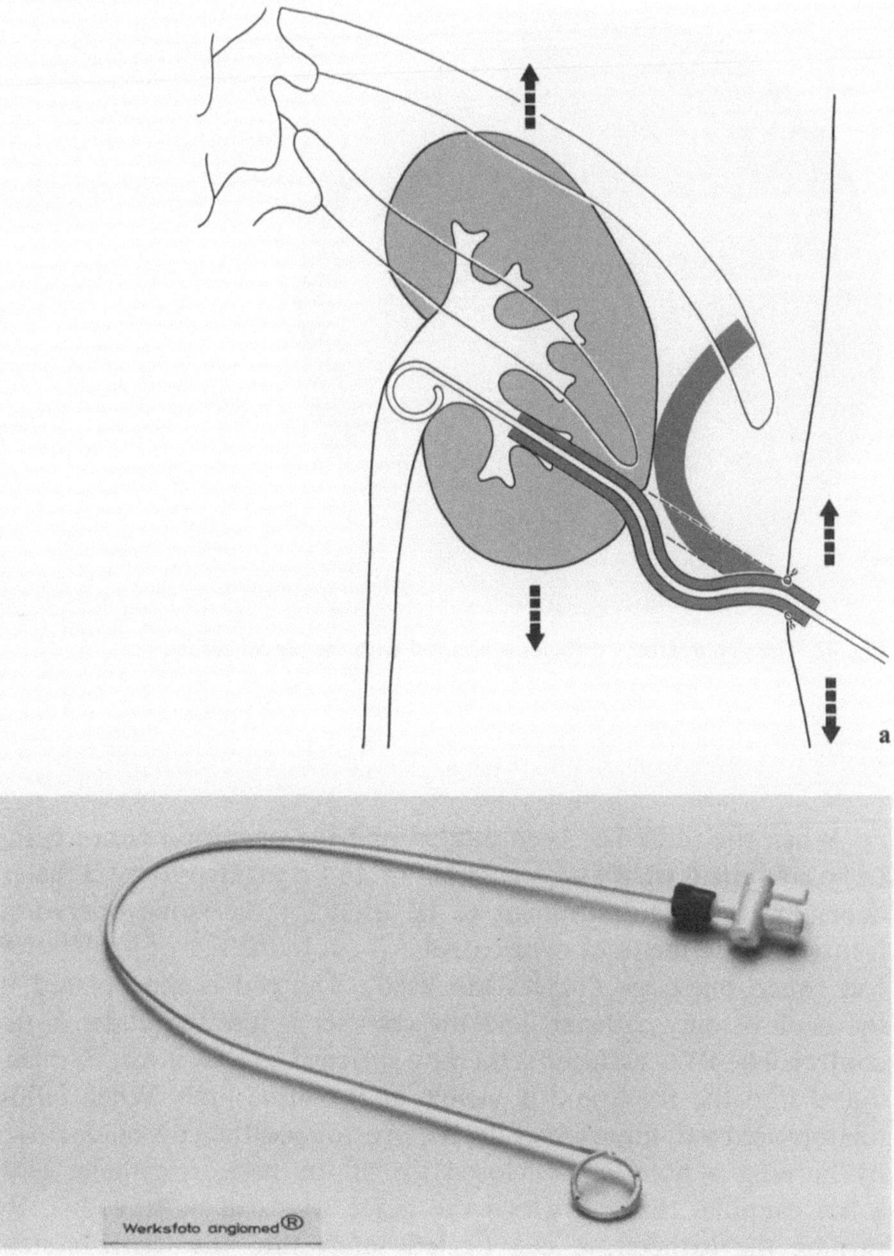

Fig. 41. a To keep the nephrostomy catheter from slipping out of the track when the kidney moves, it is secured with a pigtail catheter. The pigtail catheter lies freely in the nephrostomy catheter providing a telescope-like extension of the catheter. **b** When a pigtail catheter is placed in the nephrostomy catheter, the valve at the end of the pigtail catheter is cut off and put in the tube of the drainage bag. It must not be fixed to the nephrostomy catheter

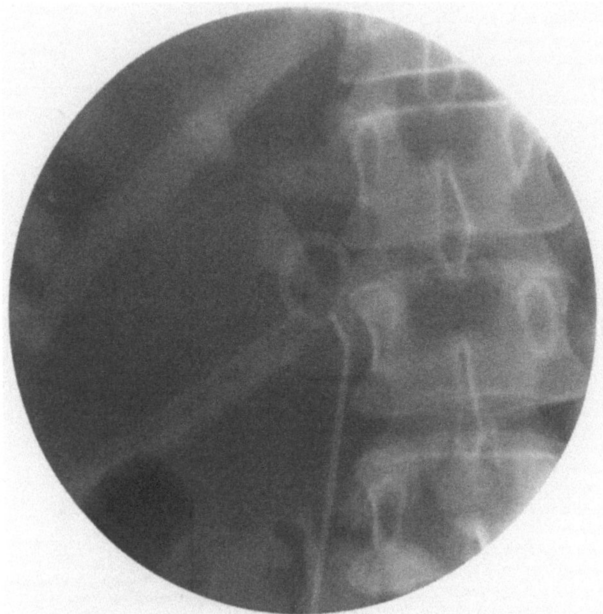

Fig. 42. The nephrostomy catheter is secured with the pigtail catheter

When the track has been dilated and the operation is not going to be continued right away, a 24 Fr. or 26 Fr. nephrostomy catheter, depending on the instrument to be used for the stone operation, is inserted into the track. The catheter is cut to the size of a dilatation rod (when telescope dilators are used). The rod is then placed in the nephrostomy catheter, and the catheter is inserted under X-ray control. The PVC catheter is thereby stiffened so that it can be introduced into the track and is visible at the same time. When teflon dilators are used, insertion of the nephrostomy catheter is made easier by burning a hole in the closed tip of the nelaton catheter with a hot cannula, through which the guide wire can be threaded. By turning the catheter, it can be led safely into the cavity system (Fig. 40a).

Nephrostomy catheters used to keep the track open should be made of material that is rejected by the body, such as PVC or rubber. Such material quickly effects a stable percutaneous track due to the strong defense reaction of the body. Materials such as silicon or polyurethane are tolerated by the body and are thus unsuited for this purpose. They should only be used if the operation is to be carried out in one session (Fig. 40b).

Fixating the nephrostomy catheter poses a problem, particularly if the patient is adipose. Movement of the kidney when the patient breathes and the mobility of the skin cause the tip of the catheter, which is sewn to the skin, to slip out. This problem can be solved by advancing a pigtail catheter through the nephrostomy catheter into the renal cavity system. The other end of the pigtail catheter, which is cut, lies freely in the nephrostomy catheter. The pigtail catheter thus effects both a stiffening of the nephrostomy catheter and a telescope-like extension of the catheter. Even if the tip of the nephrostomy catheter completely leaves the kidney, one can easily find the track again via the pigtail catheter (Figs. 41a, b; 42).

K. The Percutaneous Operation of Kidney Stones

The percutaneous operation of kidney stones can be carried out in one or more sessions.

1. Operation in one Session

An operation in one session consists of puncturing the kidney, dilating the track, and inserting the sheath of the pyeloscope into the kidney to remove the stone (Fig. 43). The advantage of this procedure is that the patient only has to undergo a single operation and can be released relatively soon afterwards. The disadvantages are that the operation is sometimes lengthy and that in some cases there can be freshly coagulated blood in the kidney due to the dilatation and puncture, which obstructs visualization. Another disadvantage is that it is impossible to remove the pyeloscope from the percutaneous track (in order to extract large stone fragments that are as large as the track, for example,) without inserting safety guide wires. This can be very time-consuming. Furthermore, if a large fragment slips out of the basket into the non-stable track, the stone disappears into the fatty tissue and is never found again. Although the stone can usually stay there without causing any damage, it later disturbs the "cosmetics" of the X-ray.

The safety wire is inserted either through the special dilator from the telescope dilator set or in the following manner: after the outer sheath of the pyeloscope has been inserted and the dilators removed, 2 (or more) Seldinger wires are placed into the kidney through the empty sheath. The sheath is then removed and, after the obturator is inserted, a wire is threaded through its central hole. The sheath can then be easily re-led into the kidney (Fig. 44a, b).

The Amplatz sheath represents a so-called temporary track which is advanced through a dilatation rod and left as a track between the skin and the renal pelvis (Fig. 45). This makes the pyeloscope moveable. The disadvantage of the Amplatz sheath, however, is that

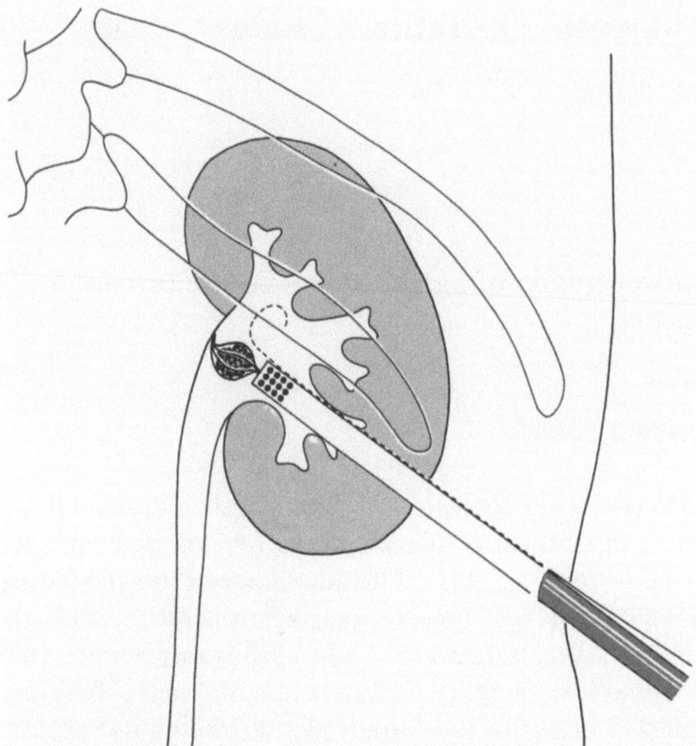

Fig. 43. If stones are to be extracted in toto through a newly laid track with the instrument, a guide wire must first be laid parallel to the pyeloscope so that the way back to the kidney can be found

it cannot be widened if, for example, stones that are larger than the sheath itself have to be extracted. Furthermore, the track has to be dilated 2 Fr. to 3 Fr. more than the usual width, which causes the destruction of kidney tissue. It does not take long before 30 Fr. are reached. Instead of the sheath, I suggest using larger instruments, which offer better optics and better handling.

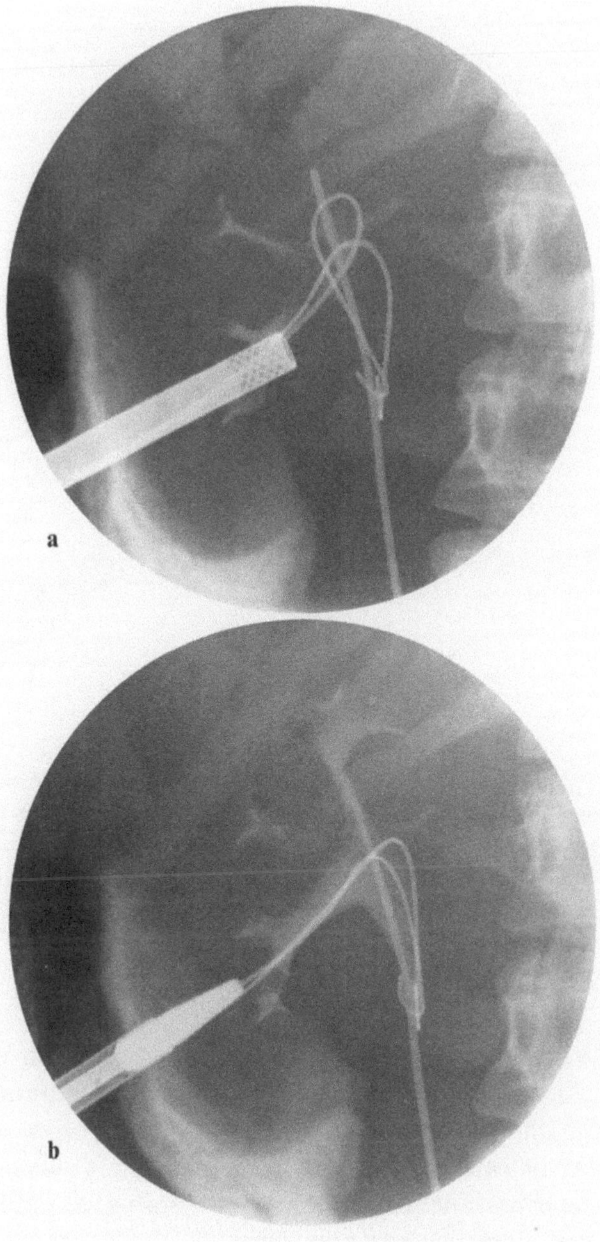

Fig. 44a, b. Inserting a safety wire into a newly laid track parallel to the pyeloscope is done by passing 2 wires through the empty outer sheath and advancing the outer sheath over one of the 2 wires. This is guided by a hollow obturator

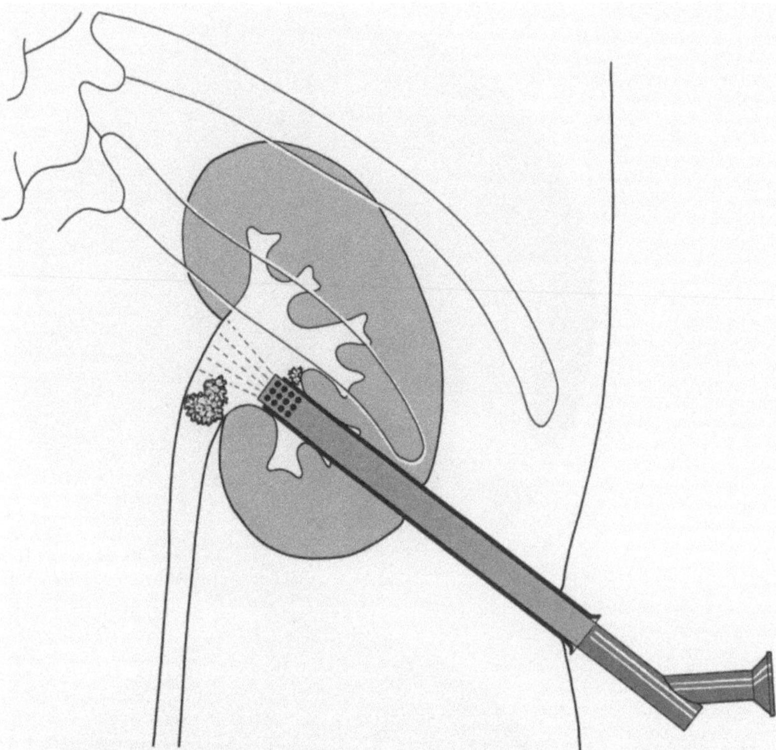

Fig. 45. The Amplatz sheath provides a "stable track" for the duration of the operation. Small stone fragments easily become hidden under the sheath

2. Operation Using an Established Track

When the stone operation is carried out in more than one session using the same track, the track becomes granulated and stable, allowing the pyeloscope to be removed as often as desired without the aid of safety wires. As early as 3 to 4 days after it has been laid, the percutaneous track becomes stable, resembling a tube. Particularly if there is scar adherence to the lateral abdominal wall from a previous operation, an analgetic, stable track developes all the way to the kidney, which is ready to be used 2 days after it is laid. The track is generally free of blood. Any blood clots in the kidney are so firm that they can be extracted whole with a small forceps. Large stone fragments or entire stones are removed through the track in the same way (Fig. 46). Even a calculus that is slightly larger than

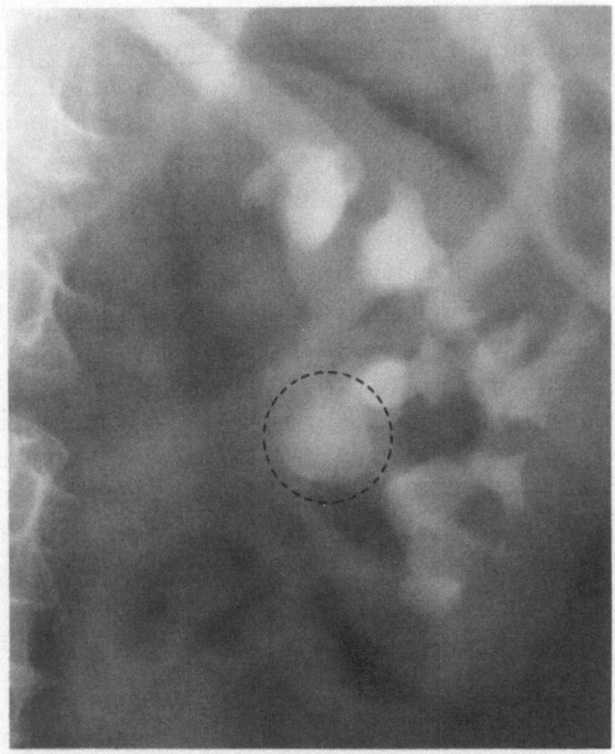

Fig. 46. A granulated percutaneous track, about 4 days old, is stable and elastic enough to allow the extraction of even large stones. Here a $17 \times 16 \times 11$ mm large stone that was removed through an 8 mm track. A notch was additionally cut into the skin

the track can pass through it, since the track can be dilated, particularly if a cross-shaped notch has been cut into the fascia lombodorsalis with the double blade knife. The actual stone removal proceeds more quickly because safety measures, such as additional wires, are not necessary to find the track again. There is no real disadvantage for the patient, since both dilatation and stone removal are carried out under local anesthesia. For the removal of staghorn stones, only stable, previously laid tracks are used, as it is essential that the pyeloscope be able to switch tracks. Another reason for carrying out the percutaneous operation in several sessions is that the operation schedule can be better organized. Puncture and dilatation are usually carried out rather quickly, especially if the surgeon has had a lot of practice, so that the time involved is roughly 15 to 30 min. Medium-sized urological departments should have no problem fitting these short procedures into their operating schedule. And the time needed for the actual removal of the stone can be calculated according to its size and the position of the track.

The removal of kidney stones in one surgical session, but without using an Amplatz sheath and safety wires, is ideal for small calculi of the renal pelvis and in the upper ureter, particularly for stones that can be removed directly through the sheath. It is not conducive, however, for operations on dilated, pyelonephritic, or pyonephrotic kidneys because it can result in a severe pyelorenal reflux with subsequent chills and fever. In such cases, puncture and dilatation must always be carried out first and, after the congestion has been relieved and antibiotic treatment has been carried out, the patient must be free from fever for several days before the actual removal of the stone can be performed.

a) Small Pelvic Stones

The percutaneous removal of a small pelvic stone no larger than a hazlenut is the ideal operation for the beginner at this technique. The track is first dilated and granulated. In the second session, the pyeloscope is advanced towards the stone and grasps it with the basket. The basket is then closed tightly and extracted together with the pyeloscope. A nephrotomy catheter is inserted and the operation is over.

The use of Dormia baskets in the renal cavity system is not recommended in every case. These baskets have a long, hard, soldered tip, which makes it impossible for the basket to lie directly on the renal pelvis. This not only makes it difficult to get hold of the stone, but also risks tearing the kidney with the hard tip. The soft baskets, such as the ones used for the flexible endoscope, are better suited. Although they too have a soldered tip, they have soft, meshed wires that bend at the least bit of pressure.

b) Stones in the Upper Ureter

The importance of an accurately laid percutaneous track, particularly in the case of a calculus in the upper ureter, has already been stated. After the pyeloscope has entered the ureter, the stone can often be seen jutting out. It is then grasped with the forceps and carefully and slowly pulled out. In such a case, the operation goes just as quickly as the operation on renal calculi. Occasionally, however, a stone is found that has been in the ureter for a long time and is impacted, making it impossible to reach it with the forceps. Care must be taken that an uncontrolled movement does not force the stone any further into the ureter. It is also dangerous to insert a Dormia basket or a flexible basket next to the stone impacted in the upper ureter because the basket can perforate the ureter. In such cases, it is advisable to insert a ureteral catheter retrograde into the ureter prior to the operation and to try to force the stone into the renal pelvis, where one can get at it easily. If the stone refuses to be moved and only the tip of the ureteral catheter projects into the renal pelvis, one can try tying a loop to the other end of the catheter and pulling both the catheter and the loop upwards. Some calculi in the upper ureter can be removed this way.

Stones in the upper ureter can be far more problematic than stones in the renal pelvis. For this reason, extreme caution is mandatory. Basically, however, it can be said that any calculus in the upper ureter that can be seen can be removed. This also applies to dilated ureters, into which it is sometimes possible to get far down with the flexible endoscope (Fig. 47a, b).

c) Large Pelvic Stones

A renal pelvic stone too large to be removed in one piece through the track can be disintegrated by various means. A stone the size of a cherry, for example, can be cut up into several pieces with the punch instrument and extracted directly. This is also a very quick procedure. Disintegrating renal pelvic stones by ultrasound is possible in most cases, however, it can be very time-consuming if the calculus is hard. The ultrasound method itself is not dangerous and, according to reports on the application of the technique to date, damage to the renal pelvic wall is minimal. The danger, however, is that the ultrasound probe can shove the stone causing it to become impacted or to tear the kidney.

An effective and fast method is the electrohydraulic disintegration of renal pelvic stones. It is also a reliable method, provided the same criteria are used as for its application for the bladder. The method must always be carried out under visual control and the continuous flow of water around the stone must be sufficient to pick up the

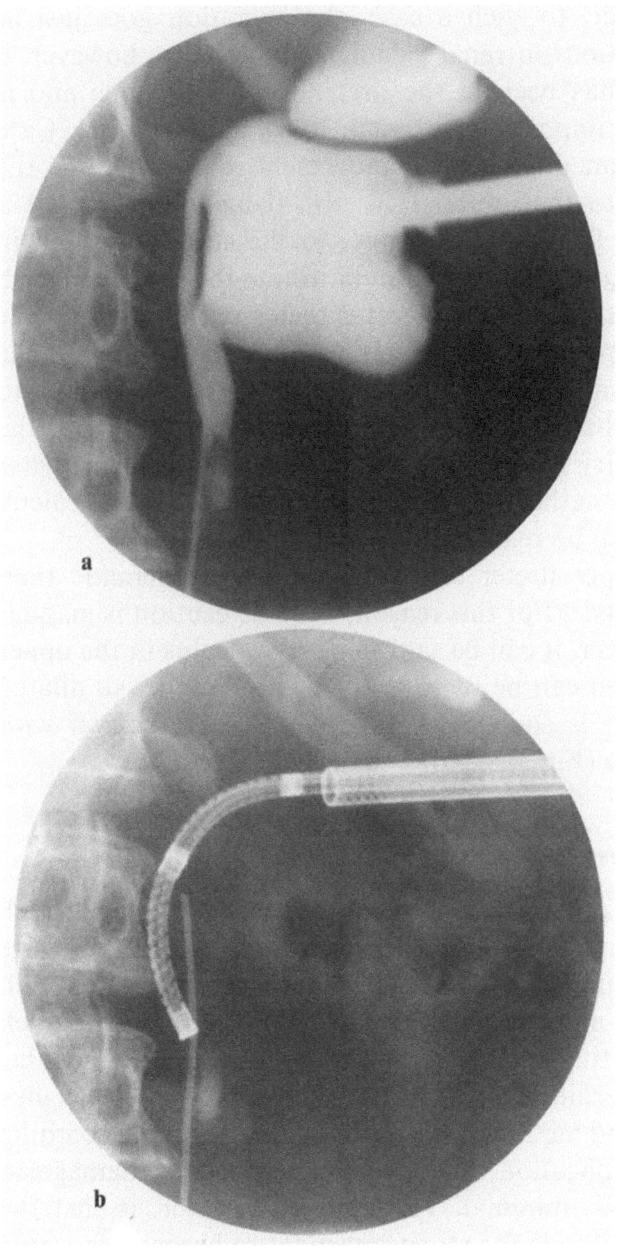

Fig. 47a, b. Large stone in the upper ureter, for the most part asymptomatic, had been in this position for 6 months and was not extractable. Disintegration by electro-hydraulic shockwaves by means of a 4 Fr. probe in the fiberscope (see also color plate III, N)

shockwaves and to absorb the energy. Care must be taken that the tip of the probe is not brought too close to the renal pelvic wall.

Large stones can generally be disintegrated with the electrohydraulic probe and the fragments extracted individually. Stone gravel is usually removed by suction (see section on staghorn stone). In operations, in which the stone first has to be desintegrated before it can be removed, a balloon catheter or a thick ureteral catheter should always be placed in the ureter to prevent stone fragments from sliding down into the ureter and blocking it (Fig. 48a–d).

d) Calyceal Stones

A calyceal stone can be removed easily when the track passes through the respective calyx towards the renal pelvis. Stones in other calyces are removed with the fiberscope. The idea here is to make a renal pelvic stone out of a calyceal stone, so that the actual manipulation of the stone is done in the renal pelvis. Using the fiberscope, the different calyces are illuminated and the stones are extracted with the aid of a loop or baskets. Drawing stones out of cystically dilated calyces into the kidney is difficult, since the fiberscope is usually not thin enough to pass through the narrow calyx neck. In this case, it is wise to split the calyx neck in the longitudinal direction of the kidney with a diathermy knife (danger of bleeding!) or the flexible scissors. The stone can then either be rinsed out or drawn out with a basket. An "active loop" is presently being developed for the extraction of impacted stones, which will make it possible to push a wire of the loop in between the stone and the calyx.

Occasionally a calyceal stone lies so close to the track that it is impossible to enter the calyx, even with the flexible endoscope bent back. Using the rigid pyeloscope and the scissors with the outside cutting edge, it is possible to get directly into the calyx through the track wall and the calyx wall and to proceed towards the stone with the pyeloscope. The stone can then be pushed into the renal pelvis or one can try to pull it out. There is surprisingly little bleeding with this procedure, perhaps because chronic calculosis in this region causes heavy scarring and vessel destruction (Figs. 49–50).

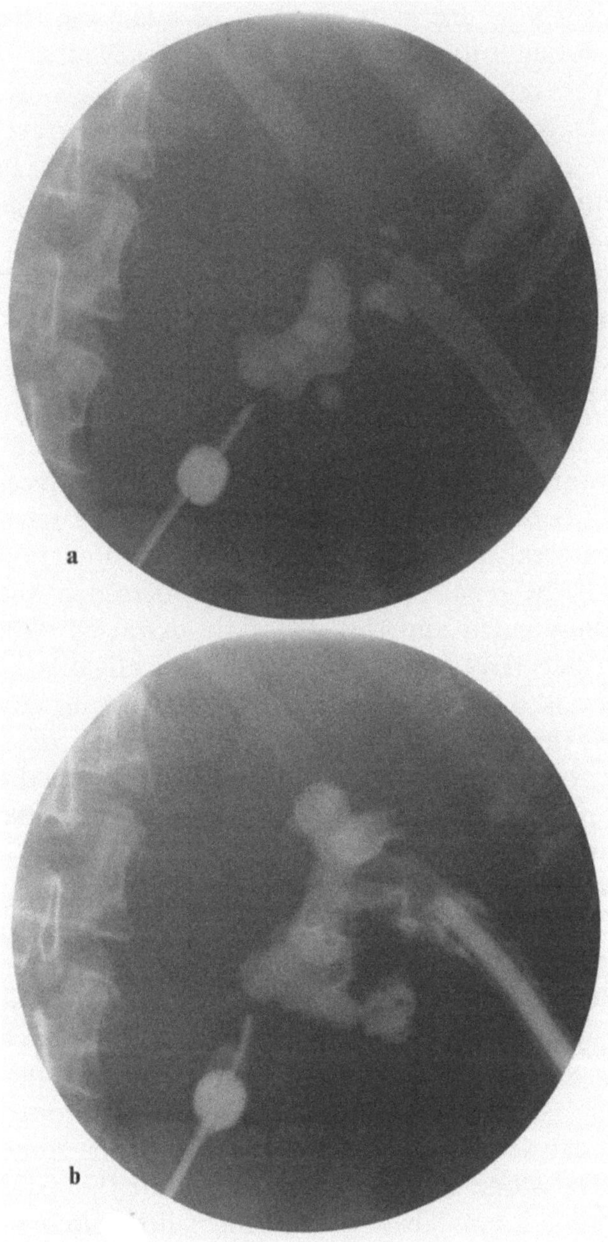

Fig. 48 a–d. Percutaneous track leads directly to the stone in the middle calyx group. After removal of the calyx stone, the large pelvic stone is electrohydraulically disintegrated. Ureter blocked with balloon catheter

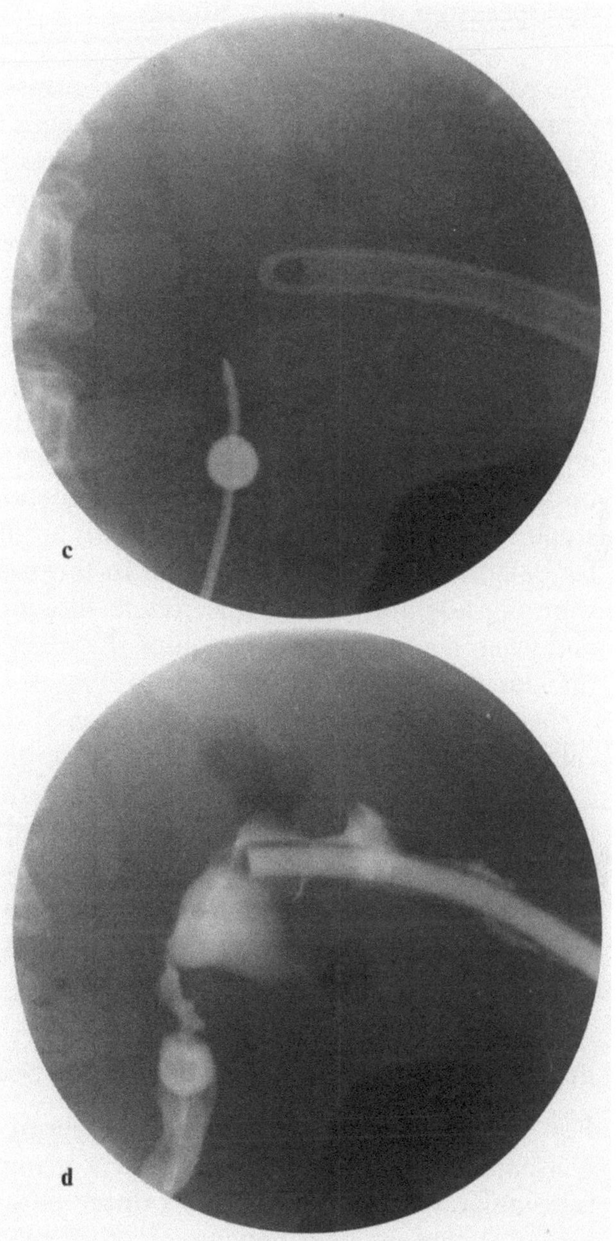

3. Operation of Staghorn Stones

The percutaneous removal of staghorn stones without a doubt represents the technical limits of the percutaneous method. It also reveals, however, the change that surgical principles regarding the operation of kidney stones have undergone. The surgeon is no longer forced to ensure that the kidney be completely free of stones at the end of surgery, since the operation can be interrupted at any time, it can be carried out in several sessions, and it can be repeated later on with no difficulty. The decision whether or not to remove all the stones is made for each individual case, based on the surgical indication, the condition of the kidney, and the surgical risk of the patient (Fig. 52a–d). To give an example: a kidney has been operated on several times and now harbors one staghorn stone and numerous stones in the calyces. In my opinion, it would be a mistake to aim for complete removal of the stones in this case if the creatinine level were considerably raised, the iodine hippuran clearance very low, and when percutaneous removal of the main stone alone could keep the kidney free from infection for 1–2 years.

Although the percutaneous operation of staghorn stones is technically difficult, I still prefer it to open surgical methods. It can be carried out in more than one session, relatively little parenchyma is destroyed, and qualitatively it can be considered a sort of microsurgery.

Particularly the last point is likely to show in a few years that this method, more than open surgery, has reduced the incidence of recurrent stones (Fig. 53a–d).

a) Disintegration of Stones: Irrigation and Suction Technique

For the percutaneous removal of staghorn stones, the first track is usually laid through the lower calyx group. From here the stone is disintegrated and the fragments rinsed out. Depending on the location of further stone fragments or other calculi, 1 or 2 more tracks are laid through the middle and upper calyx groups. Tracks through the upper pole are dangerous because they can cause damage to neighboring organs. Tangential penetration of the parenchyma results in injury to numerous vessels, which causes severe bleeding. The actual disintegration of the calculus is done – as has already been discussed – either with the ultrasound instrument or with the

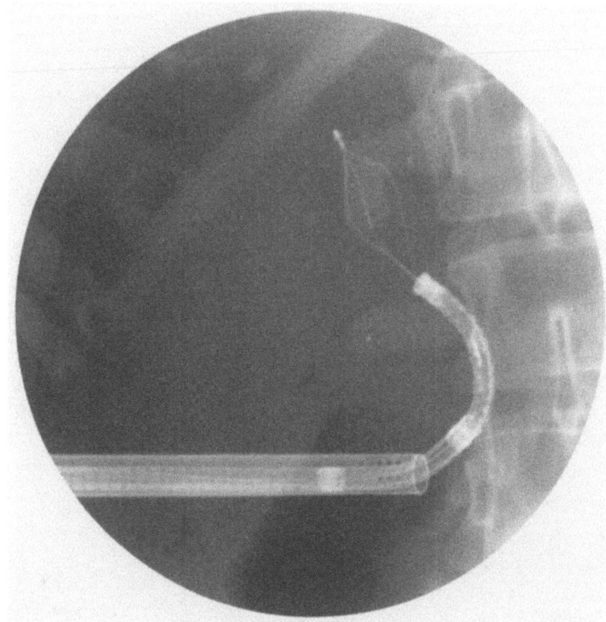

Fig. 49. A stone is extracted from the upper pole and shifted to the renal pelvis where it can be manipulated

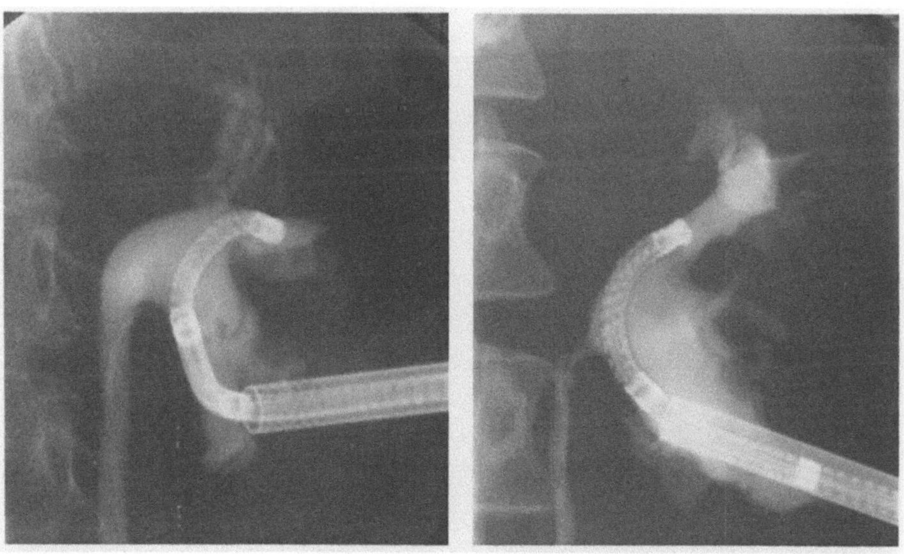

Fig. 50   **Fig. 51**

Fig. 50. Inspection of the middle calyces through the flexible fiberscope

Fig. 51. Inspection of the upper calyx group through the flexible fiberscope. Extending the tip of the endoscope solves the distance problem

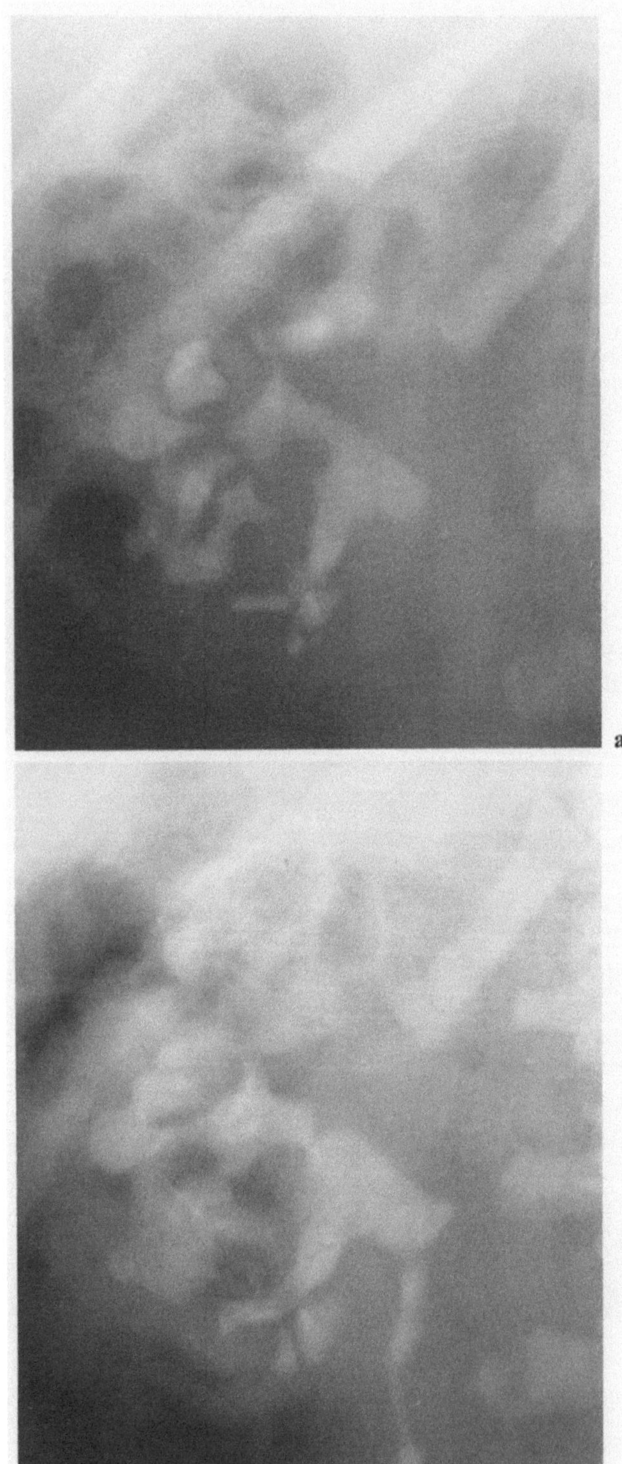

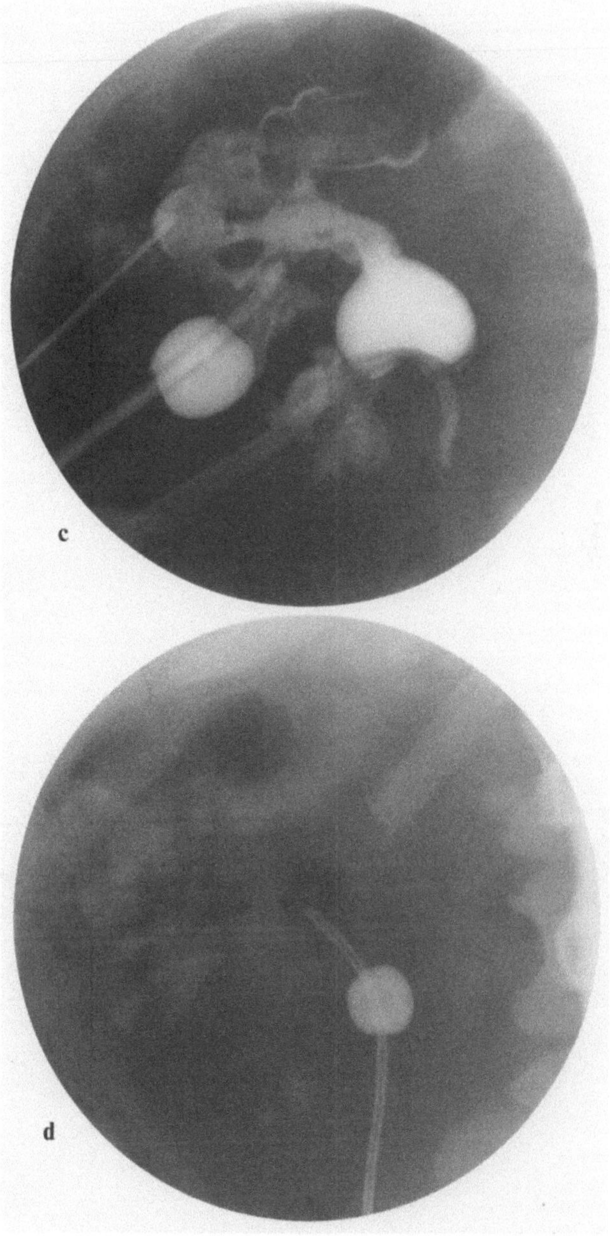

Fig. 52a–d. 53 year old man, the same single kidney operated on 4 times, the last time was a year ago. Percutaneous operation of a large pelvic stone with numerous enclosed calyceal stones. It was not possible to remove all of the calyceal stones without endangering the kidney

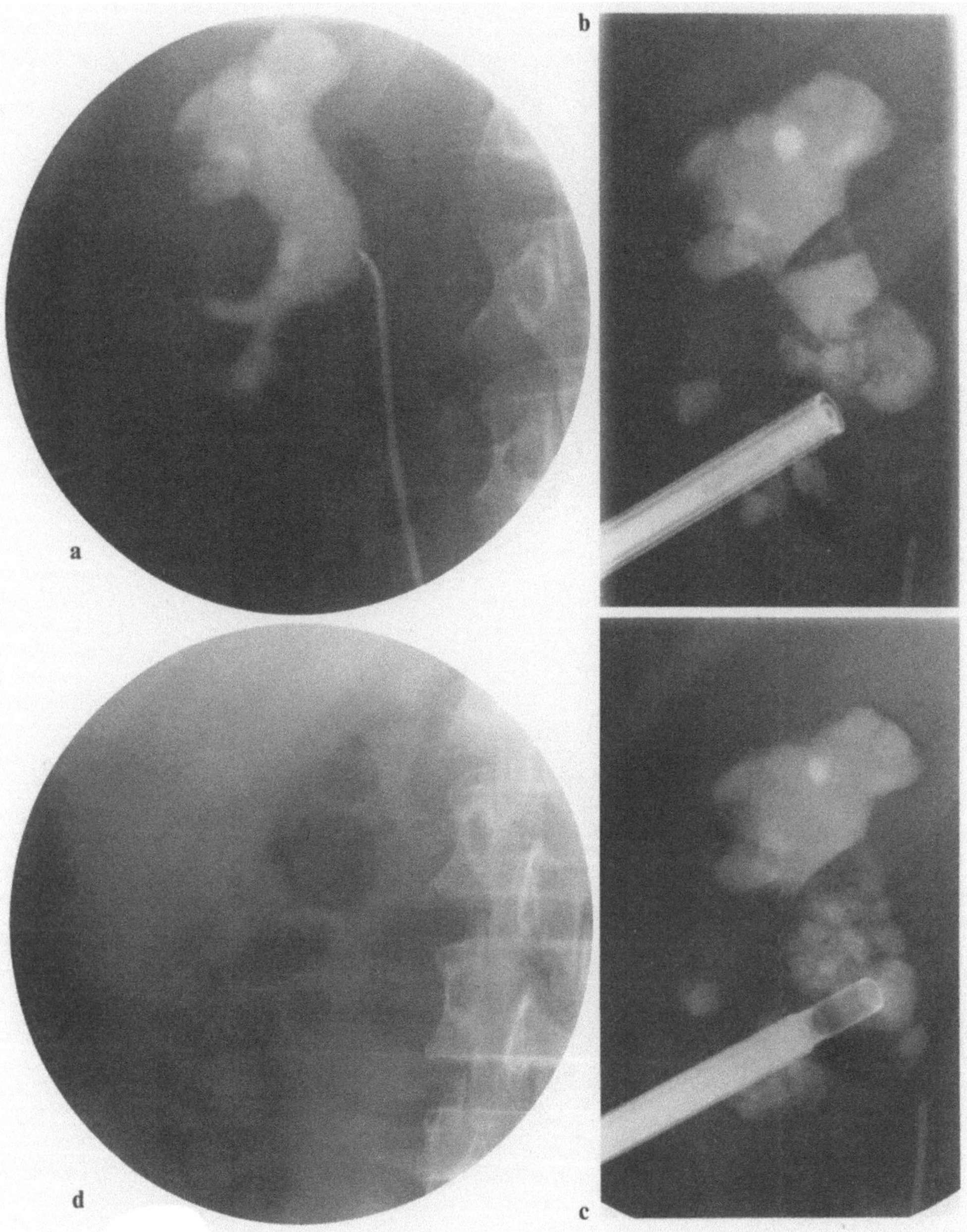

Fig. 53a–d. Very hard, calcified cystine recurrent stone was disintegrated by electro-hydraulic shockwaves and ultrasound. This was done in 4 surgical sessions and under local anesthesia

electrohydraulic device. Large stone fragments are extracted directly through the track, in some cases together with the instrument. Smaller fragments can be rinsed out through the sheath using the rinsing attachment instead of the lens. Calculi the size of the inner sheath can be removed in the following way: a constant flow of irrigant enters the kidney through the outer sheath. Intermittent pressing of the suction regulation valve causes the renal pelvis to move like a pump. The stone fragments whirl around and, after they are drawn through the sheath by suction, collect in a balloon flask. Small pieces of the calculi are removed under direct supervision: the irrigant again flows through the outer sheath but suction is done through the instrument channel. The quality of vision is relatively poor but good enough to allow adequate control (Fig. 54a–c).

To disintegrate large calculi, a combination of electrohydraulic energy with the ultrasound probe can be used. After the stone is quickly destroyed and the larger fragments rinsed out, the instrument destroys the small pieces and sucks them out like a vacuum cleaner.

b) Laying a New Track

To lay a new track, the same procedure is used as for puncturing a non-dilated kidney. A balloon catheter is placed in the already existing track and is inflated slightly with a contrast agent to close off the track. The contrast makes the balloon catheter visible in the cavity system. The cavity system can be dilated slightly by an infusion of contrast and indigo carmine. After the best entry for the new track has been determined, puncture and dilatation can be carried out. The tracks are kept open until the end of the operation, i.e., throughout all the sessions, which allows all the tracks to be used simultaneously during one session (Fig. 55a–d).

When the operation has been completed, the nephrostomy catheter is left in place only until the bleeding has stopped. The renal fistula closes within a day when flow through the ureter is undisturbed. A urinary fistula that takes longer to close usually indicates an impairment of the urinary flow through the ureter, possibly caused by stone fragments or an edema in the ureter. In this case, a ureteral catheter should be placed retrograde in the kidney for 1 or 2 days until the leakage has stopped.

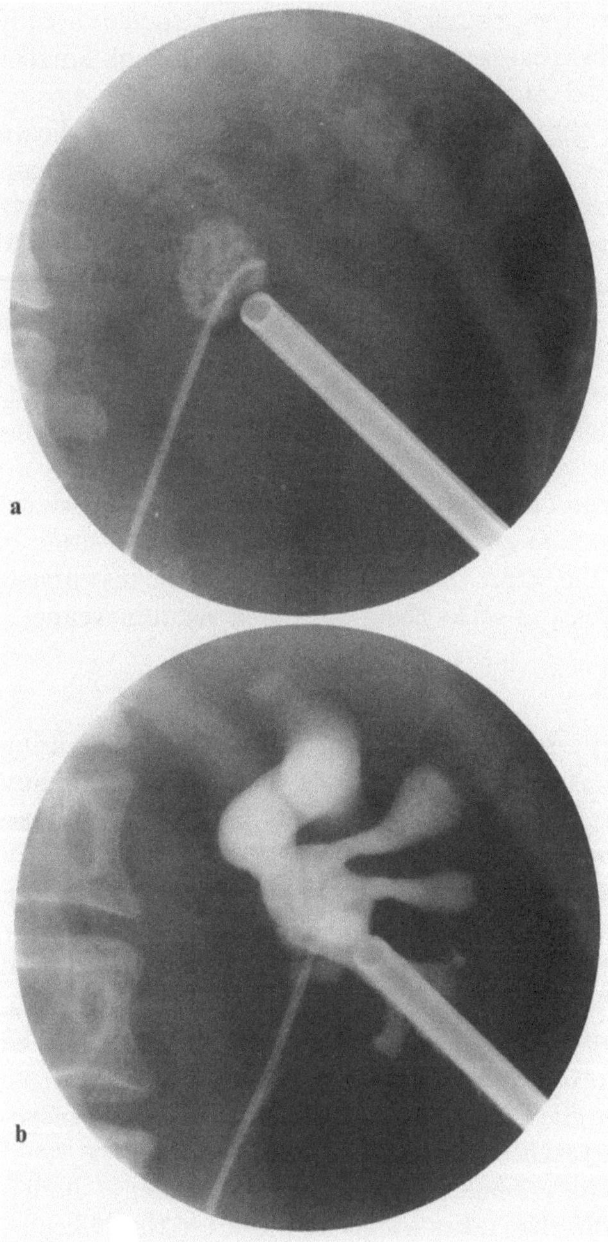

Fig. 54a–c. By reversing the direction of the irrigation, i.e. transferring irrigation to the outer sheath and suction to the inner sheath, suction can be carried out with or without direct vision, depending on the size of the stone. Intermittent activation of suction effects a pump-like movement of the cavity system

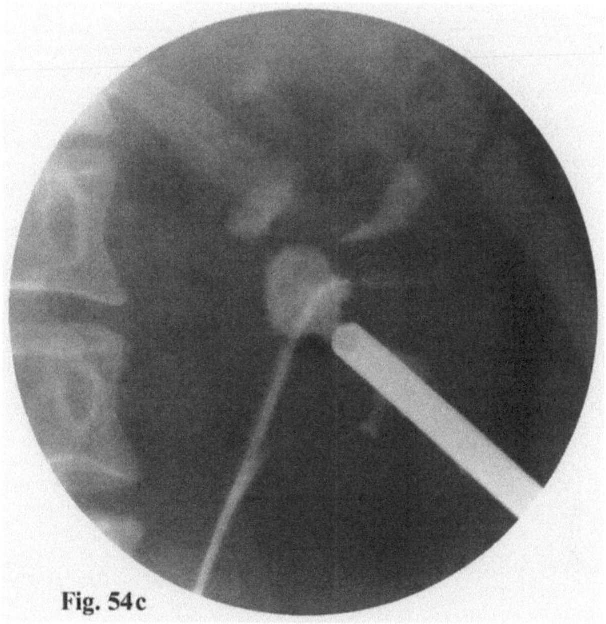

Fig. 54c

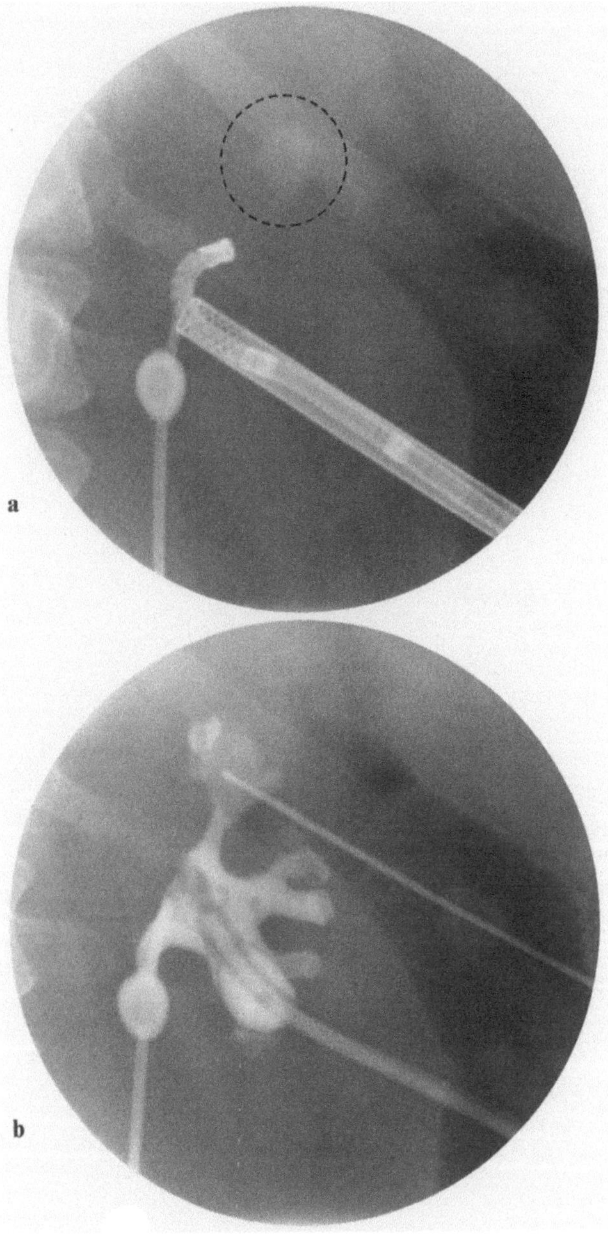

Fig. 55a–d. Laying a new track intraoperatively for a stone in the upper pole. **a** Locating the stone with the flexible fiberscope. **b** Closing off the lower end of the track with a Foley catheter and puncturing the upper calyx group. **c** Advancing a Seldinger wire. **d** Dilating the track

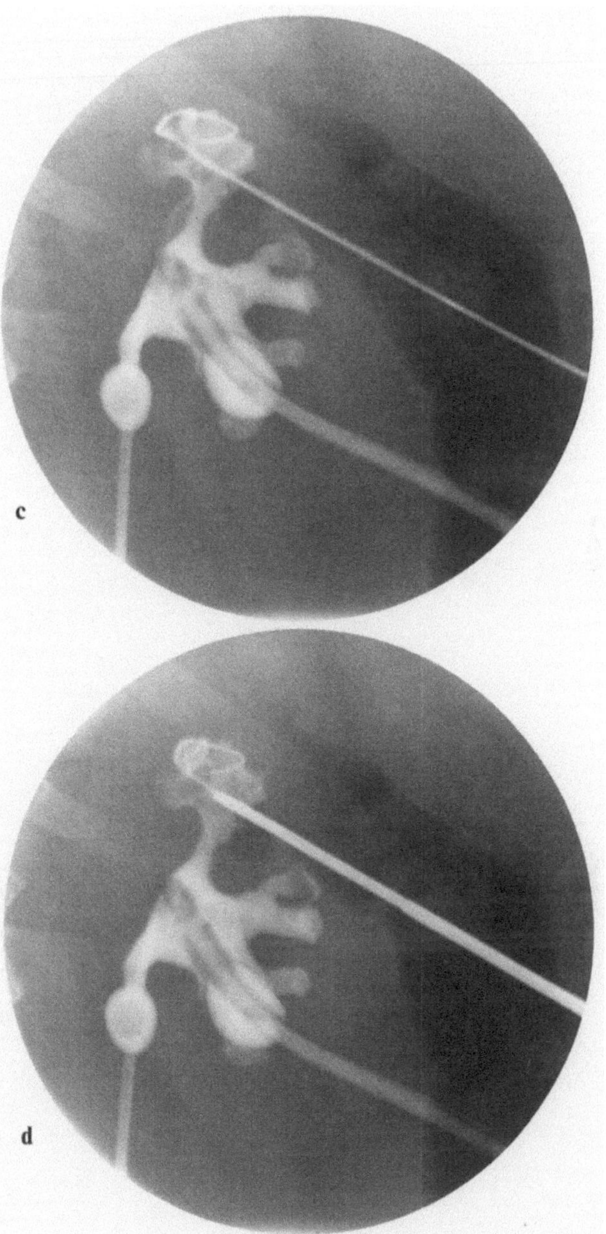

L. Complications

The most frequently arising complication during percutaneous surgery is perforation of the renal pelvis. This occurs more often during puncture and dilatation of the track and seldom during the operation itself. As long as drainage of the renal cavity system is satisfactory, there is no need to resort to open surgery (Fig. 55). After the injection of contrast, the X-ray shows extensive extravasations, some of which run a pararenal course, but most of which run paraureterally down the psoas muscle. When the puncture needle and later on the dilatation rod are securely positioned in the renal cavity system, the dilatation procedure can be terminated. If perforations occur during the actual operation, the pressure of the irrigant should be reduced as much as possible to avoid water influx similar to a transurethral resection syndrome. The operation should be interrupted and a nephrostomy catheter inserted. The wound usually heals in 2 to 3 days, at which time the operation can be continued.

Bleeding from the kidney poses a serious complication. I was confronted with this problem in 4 cases and was able to get the bleeding under control without having to rely on open surgery. The track must be free of blood clots before the source of bleeding can be found. In most cases, the bleeding comes from a large vein that has been punctured and damaged when the track was dilated. It can usually be arrested by compressing the vein, as one does with bleeding veins during prostate capsule resection. If compression with a thick nephrostomy catheter is not sufficient to stop the bleeding, the balloon of a Foley catheter can be laid directly on the site of the hemorrhage; the distance of the hemorrhage is measured from a particular point (from the middle border of the renal pelvis, for example) and inflating the balloon at this point compresses the vein. Heavy bleeding from arteries, which would necessitate special treatment, rarely occurs (Fig. 56).

When carrying out punctures through the middle and upper poles, one must be certain to check that no neighboring organ, such as the pleura, liver, spleen, or intestine, is situated in the area of the

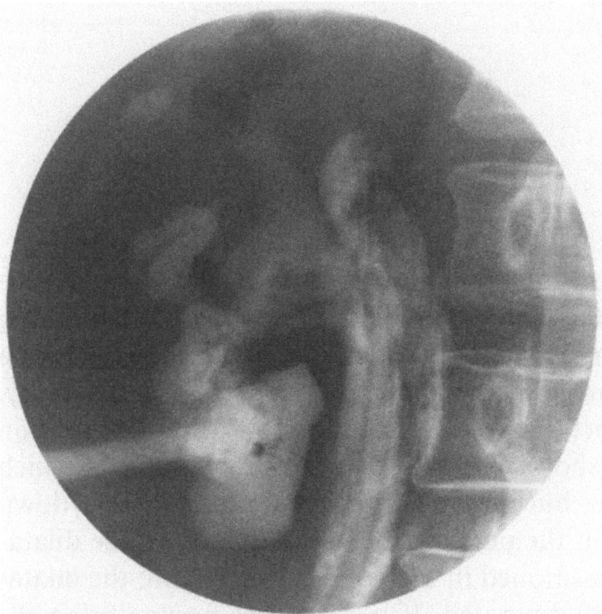

Fig. 56. Extensive parapelvine and paraureteral extravasation after pelvic perforation

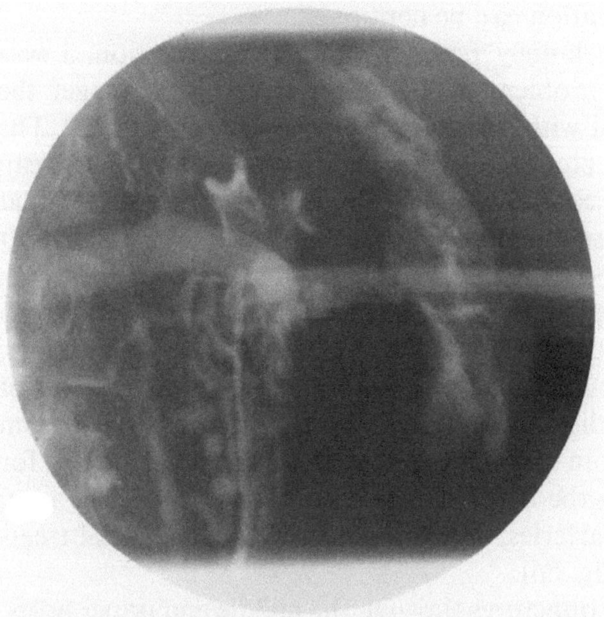

Fig. 57. Perforation of the percutaneous track into the venous system: view of capsular veins and contrast drainage through the vena renalis

puncture. This can be best established by careful ultrasonic investigation.

Nevertheless, in some cases there is going to be some damage. In our department, we had a case of a mild pneumothorax. Another patient was asymptomatic after intercostal puncture but developed bilious peritonitis after a single puncture of the upper right pole. A laparotomy performed 2 days later provided no explanation as to the site of the injury. From another hospital we heard of a postpercutaneous intraperitoneal urinary fistula. Both cases cleared up after laparotomies were carried out. We had one fatality: an extremely obese woman had been treated percutaneously for a pyonephrosis and multiple kidney stones. She died of an uncontrollable sepsis and liver failure as the result of a severe liver cirrhosis, which was not detected until autopsy.

M. Contraindications

Contraindications for the percutaneous operation include liver cirrhosis (septic complications or liver failure) and untreated blood clot disorders. Otherwise, the risk factors associated with this method are fewer than those of other operations because there is no open incision and no general anesthesia.

N. Further Indications for the Percutaneous Surgical Technique on the Kidney

1. Operations of Strictures at the Ureteropelvic Junction

If the cause of a kidney stone is a stricture at the ureteropelvic junction, it is naturally advisable to correct the obstruction after the calculus has been removed. This can be done percutaneously using the so-called "intubated ureterotomy" method developed by Davis. The stricture, depending on its position, is split open with a special flexible ureterotome or with an optical (Sachse) urethrotome (Fig. 58). After the scar tissue is completely dissected, it is essential that every fiber be separated and that a stent be applied for 3 weeks until healing is complete. For strictures at the ureteropelvic junction, an intercostal percutaneous approach should be selected to allow easy placement of the urethrotome in the ureter later on. Before the ureterotomy is performed, a ureteral catheter is inserted retrograde into the kidney with the tip of the catheter projecting out of the percutaneous track. The catheter is thus used as a stylet guide, along which the ureterotomy is carried out. The stricture is opened with the optical urethrotome until fatty tissue can be seen along the entire length of the stenosis (Fig. 59). A thick catheter of at least 9 Fr. in diameter is attached to the tip of the catheter and is drawn approximately 15 cm into the ureter to serve as a stent. At about 17 cm, holes have to be cut on the sides with the Lüer forceps to allow drainage of the renal pelvis. The stent is fixated to the catheter in the following way: the nelaton tip of the catheter is pierced with a strong needle through the uppermost hole. The thread is kept in the tip of the catheter by a large knot. The other end of the thread is left about 40 cm long and is pulled out of the urethra. A second safety thread can be attached so that in case the first thread comes loose or breaks, connection to the stent is not lost. When the stent is in proper position, the thread with the knot is pulled out and its other end is sewn to the outer opening of the percutaneous track and left indwelling for 3 weeks, at which point it can be withdrawn with ease. Only in the case of bleeding is a

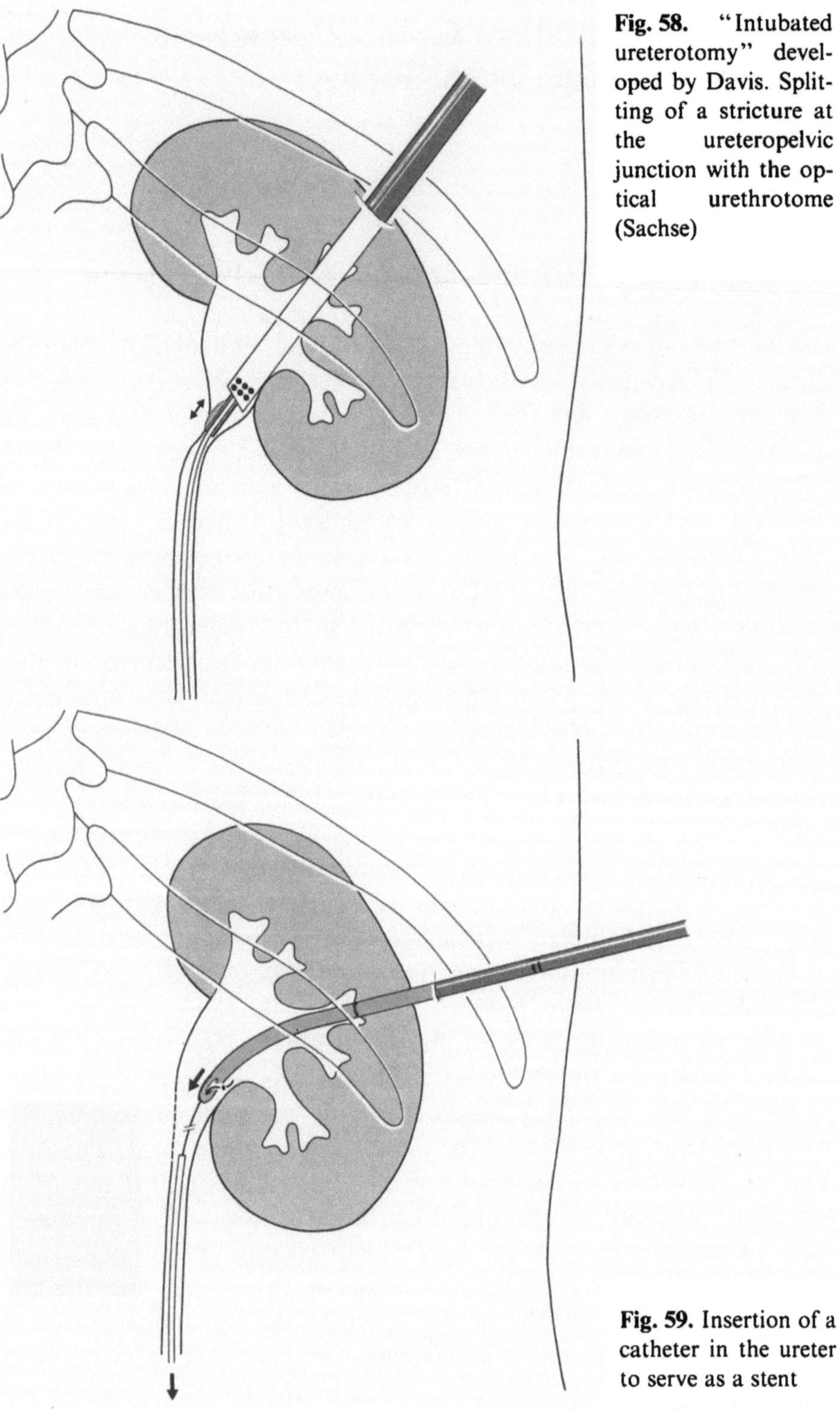

Fig. 58. "Intubated ureterotomy" developed by Davis. Splitting of a stricture at the ureteropelvic junction with the optical urethrotome (Sachse)

Fig. 59. Insertion of a catheter in the ureter to serve as a stent

nephrostomy catheter necessary for a short time after the operation. The catheter (approximately 18 Fr.) is inserted parallel to the stent (Fig. 60a–e, p. 76, 77).

A special set is being prepared which will enable the stent to be inserted under X-ray control through the percutaneous track via the ureteral catheter into the upper ureter. The ureteral catheter can then be pulled out through the stent. Here, too, the stent is fixated to the skin and left for 3 weeks.

In the case of more deeply located strictures or when the percutaneous track runs through the lower pole, it is advisable to carry out the ureterotomy with the flexible ureterotome, which is also advanced on a ureteral catheter. This procedure is controlled not by direct vision but by X-ray and the injection of a contrast agent through the instrument (Fig. 61 a, b).

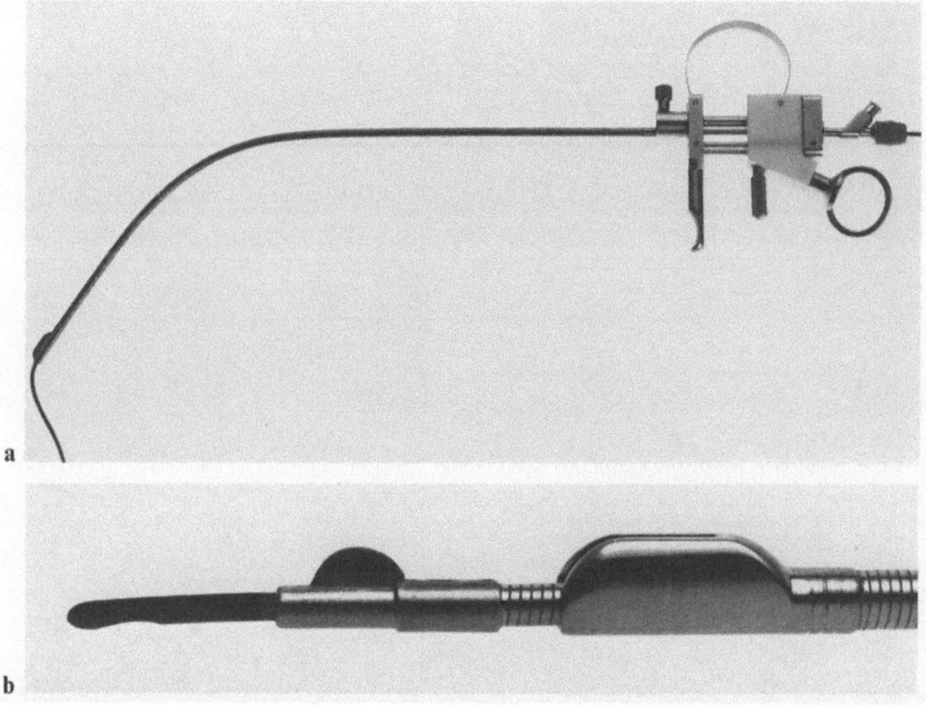

Fig. 61. a Flexible percutaneous ureterotome (no vision). The separation of the scar fibers, i.e. perforation into the fatty tissue, is controlled by X-ray after injection of contrast. **b** The ureterotome is guided along a ureteral catheter

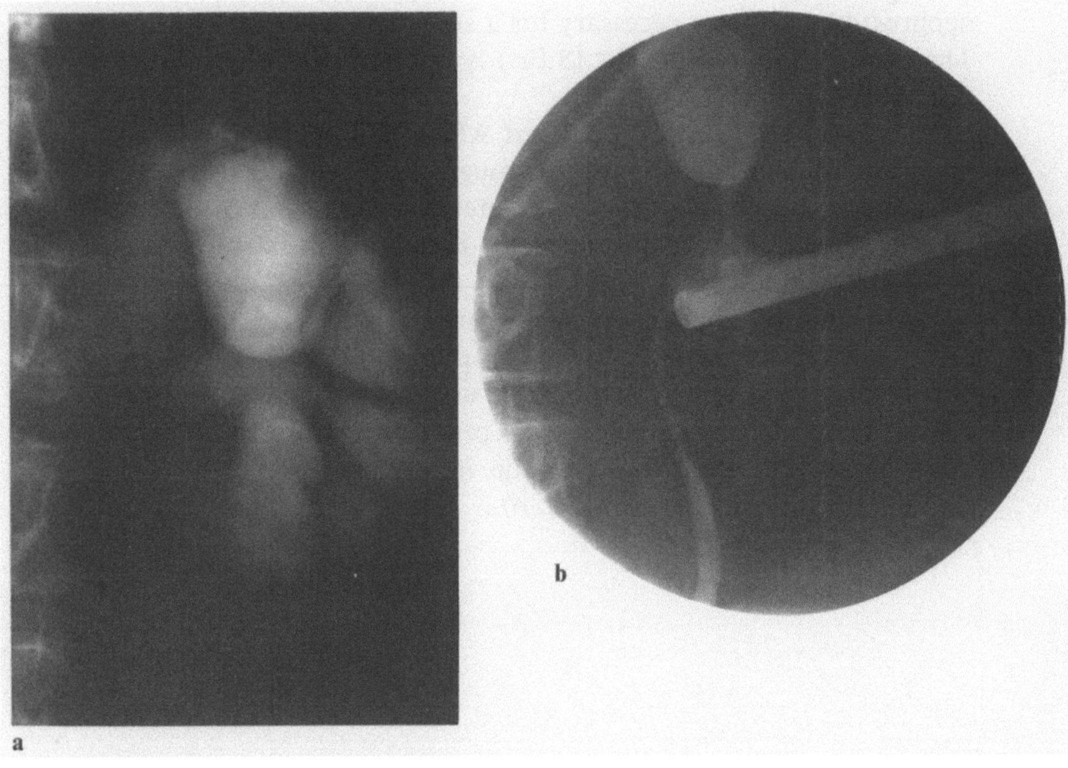

Fig. 60a–e. Percutaneous "intubated ureterotomy" after Davis. **a** Hydronephrosis caused by stricture at the ureteropelvic junction 2 years after pyelolithotomy. **b–d** Widening of the stricture on a ureteral catheter. Stent left for 3 weeks. **e** Six months later: drainage is good, the calyx is no longer plump

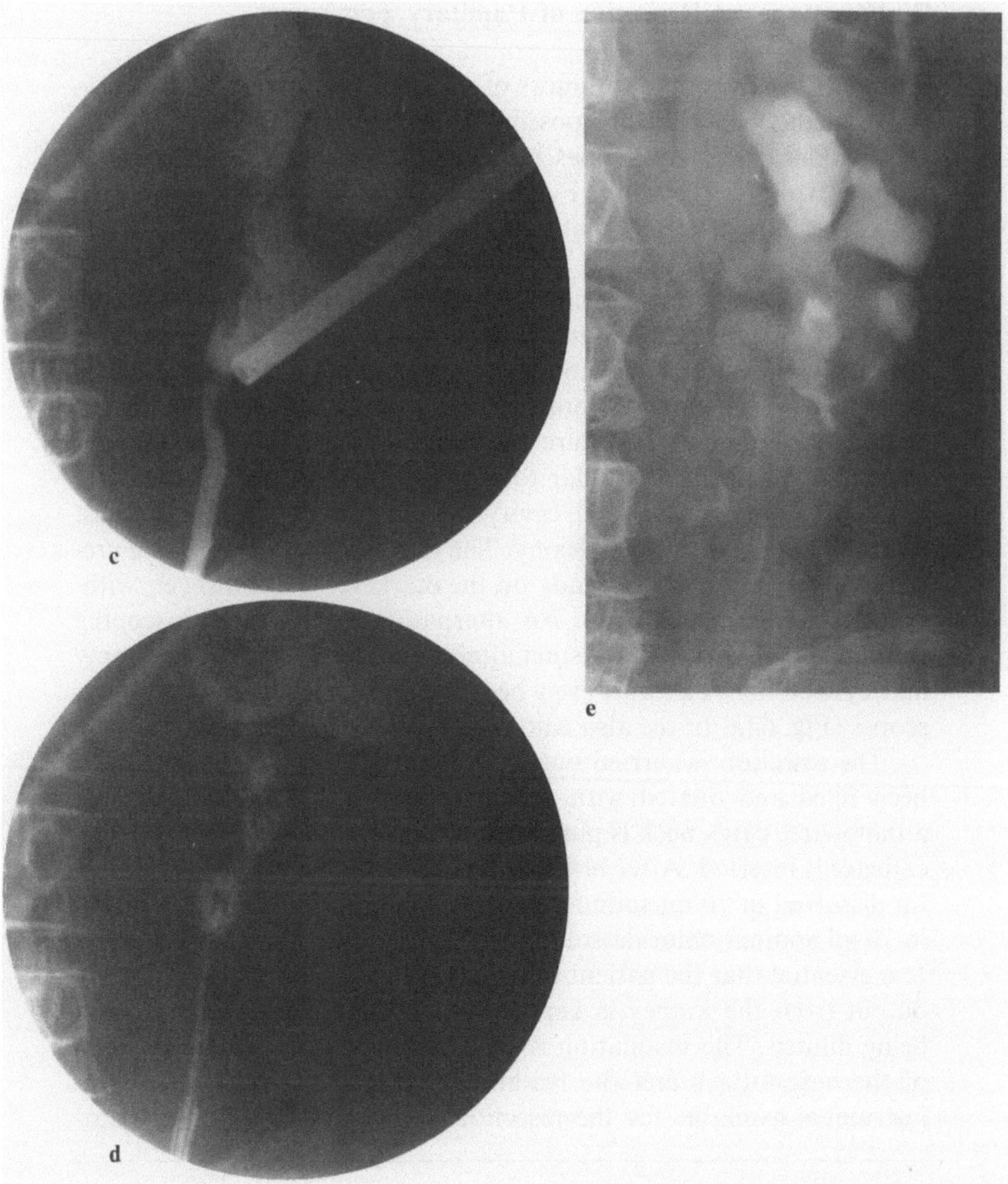

2. Percutaneous Resection of Papillary Tumors

Although the resection of tumors of the cavity system by the percutaneous method is technically possible, it is also very dangerous. Unlike the bladder, the kidney does not have a thick layer of muscle to guard it from perforation. Furthermore, the kidney is interweaved with large blood vessels that can be damaged easily if the surgical instrument goes too deep.

The indication for resection should be established individually and very critically. Candidates for the operation are elderly patients with only 1 kidney, for example, or patients with bilateral involvement, whereby 1 kidney is presumed to contain a well differentiated tumor. Nevertheless, in future the indication for the percutaneous resection will likely be similar to that for TUR in the bladder, i.e., if examination of the renal cavity system can be carried out just as well by noninvasive endoscopy. The first flexible, controllable ureterorenoscope (9 Fr.) is already on the market – still, however, without an instrument channel. An alternative would be endoscoping through a high ureter skin fistula after a unilateral nephrouterectomy and cystectomy. This can even be done with thicker, flexible fiberscopes (Fig. 62a, b; see also color plate III O, P).

The resection is carried out as follows: after the renal pelvis has been filled and dilated with a contrast agent and indigo carmine, a tumor-free calyx neck is punctured and dilated, and a nephrostomy catheter is inserted. After bleeding has been stopped, 20 mg adriblastin dissolved in 20 ml sodium chloride solution or 10 mg mitomycin in 20 ml sodium chloride solution is infused into the cavity system. It is essential that the patient have fasted for 12 h so that the urinary output from the kidney is kept low to prevent the cytostatic from being diluted. The instillation is repeated once or twice during each of the next 4 days and the resection is then carried out. The best instrument available for the resection is a continuous flow resecto-

---

Fig. 62. a 80 year old man, papillary carcinoma grade I in the right kidney. The ▷ patient has been treated for 16 years for a recurring papillary tumor in the bladder. Left nephroureterectomy 8 years ago due to urothel carcinoma grade I. Tumor in the right kidney has been known for 3 years. Local treatment with mitomycin and adriblastin with no long-term success. Tumor resection via the lower calyx neck because of recurrent bleeding. **b** Situation one year later: Patient shows no recurrent tumor and has no complaints (see also color plate III O, P)

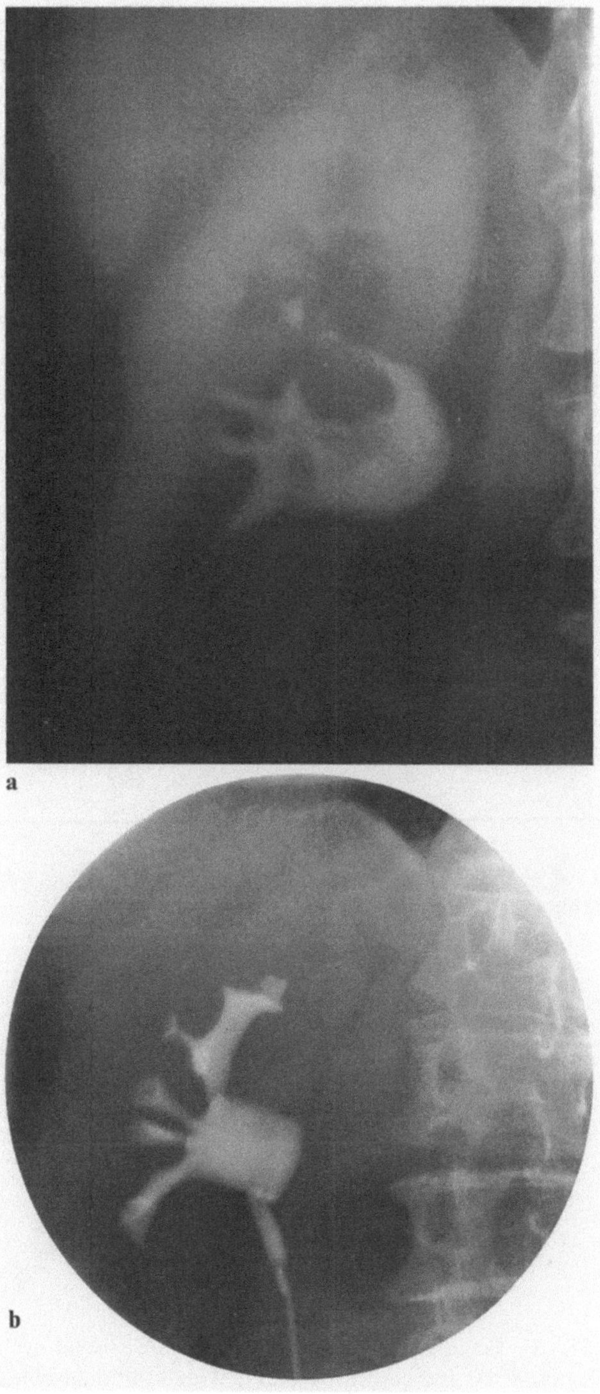

Fig. 62 a, b

sope, although a thinner instrument with thinner loops would be even better.

3. Percutaneous, Intrarenal Marsupialization of Renal Cysts

A special and rare indication for the percutaneous operation is the marsupialization of renal cysts if these cysts obstruct the flow of urine from the kidney. The aim of the operation is to join the cyst with the renal cavity system to allow continuous drainage of its content (Fig. 63; color plate III S).

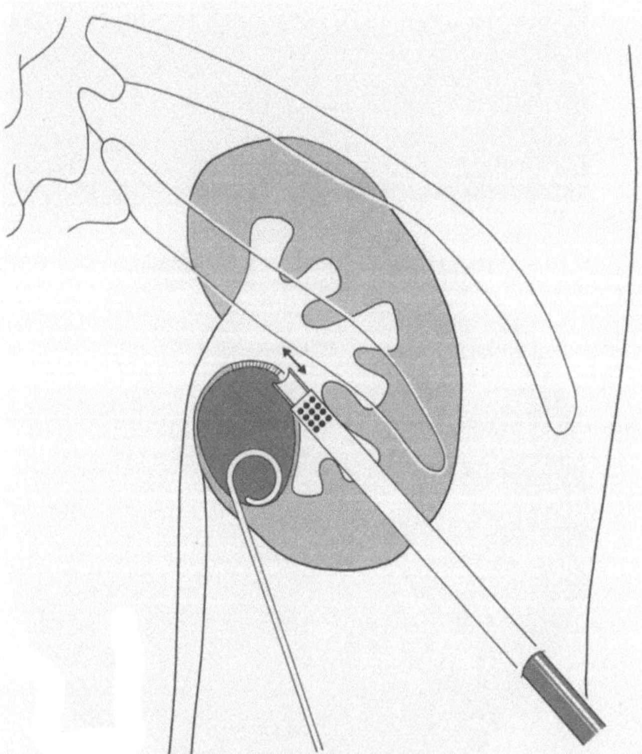

Fig. 63. Percutaneous marsupialization of a renal cyst: renal cyst is demonstrated by puncture and contrast coloring with additional blue dye. Resection of the septum void of blood vessels with the resection instrument via a suitable track. Continuous drainage into the cavity system makes the cyst part of the renal pelvis and causes it to shrink (see also color plate III, S)

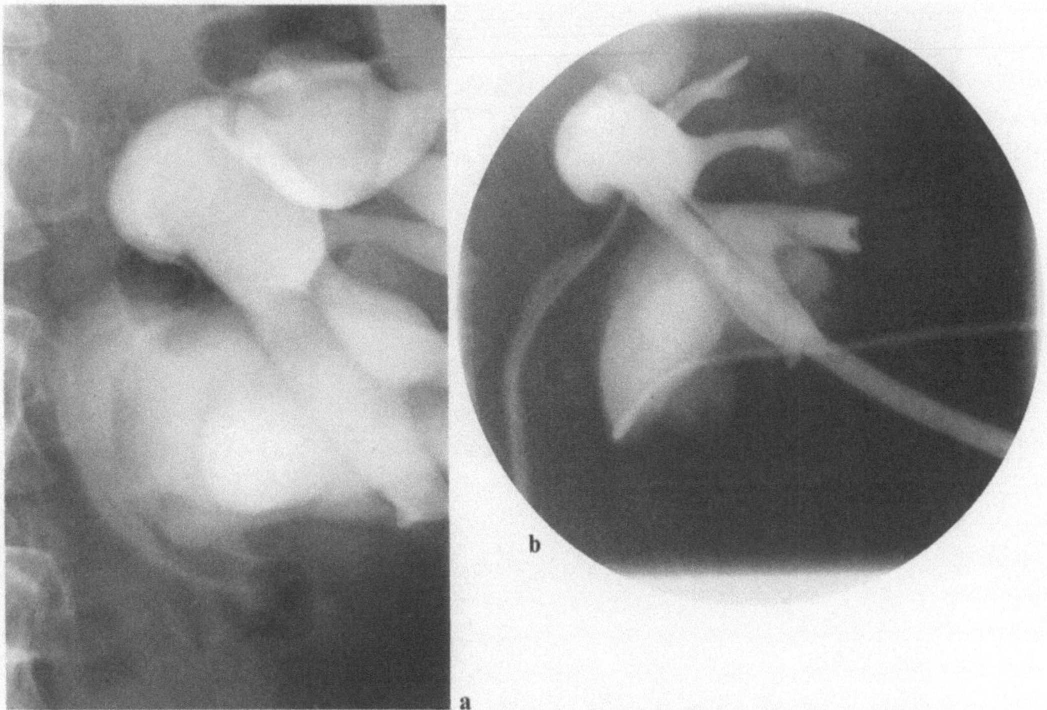

Fig. 64. a Dilated renal cavity system with upward displacement due to compression of the cyst. Medial displacement of the thin ureter. **b** A pigtail catheter lies in the cyst, a ureteral catheter is inserted retrograde in the cavity system, and a percutaneous track runs through the lower calyx

The resection of the wall between the cavity system and the renal cyst can and may only be carried out at the point where continuous compression has caused the wall to become thin and void of blood vessels. If the resectoscope enters thicker interstitial tissue, as on the rim of the cyst, it can cause damage to large blood vessels and the bleeding is extremely difficult to stop. Every surgeon is familiar with such bleeding and the problems of arresting it from open marsupialization procedures. Experience with only 4 cases up to now has shown that decompression of the cavity system or the ureter by joining the cyst to the cavity system happens quickly and that the continuous drainage of the cystic content causes the cyst to shrink rapidly and become incorporated into the renal cavity system (Fig. 64a, b).

The marsupialization is carried out in the following way: the renal cyst is punctured under ultrasound guidance and a pigtail cathe-

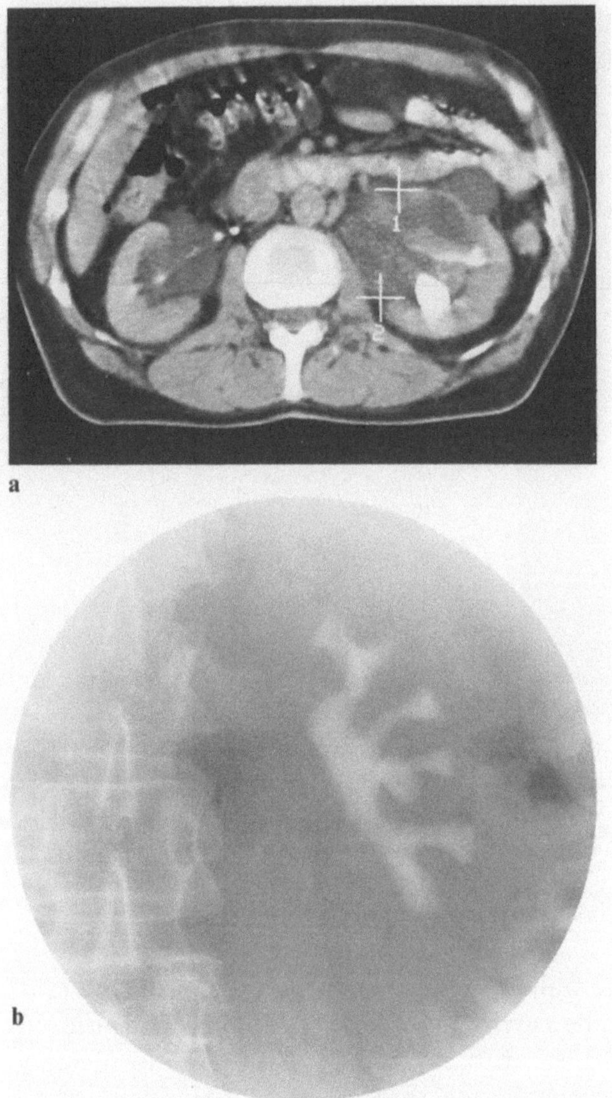

Fig. 65. a In the computertomogram – left – the large cyst; but also on the right a smaller central cyst. **b** After the wall is resected the cyst becomes part of the renal pelvis (urogram 8 weeks later)

ter is inserted. A calyx is selected as the best approach for the marsupialization, and puncture and dilatation are carried out in the manner described above. The track has to be dilated to the width of the sheath of the resectoscope to be used. After 4 to 5 days, the track is stable and the operation can begin. The renal cyst is made visible – both radiologically and later endoscopically – by an infusion of a contrast agent and blue dye. The pyeloscope is then inserted into the percutaneous track. Using an endoscopic, flexible cannula and under X-ray control, puncture is carried out in the direction of the cyst until blue dye appears. The direction of the resection is thus already established. The continuous irrigation resectoscope can now be placed in the track. The site of the puncture is widened by an incision so that the extent of the vessel-free wall can be estimated. The resection can then be performed. If necessary, tiny papillary vessels can be coagulated with a roll loop. Finally, a nephrostomy catheter is inserted and the pigtail catheter removed (Fig. 65a, b).

O. Appendix: Pyeloscopic Findings

Plate I

A Stone in a calyceal cyst which is drained into the renal pelvis through a very small neck

B Passage into the pelvis is made clear by splitting the calyx neck with a diathermy knife

C Nest of stones in a mucosa sac at the edge of a papilla

D The stones fall out of the sac after they have been grasped with the forceps via the flexible fiberscope

E Nephrocalcinosis with recurrent stone, malignant hypertonia, and hyperparathyreoidism

F Pyeloscopic view of a pyramid

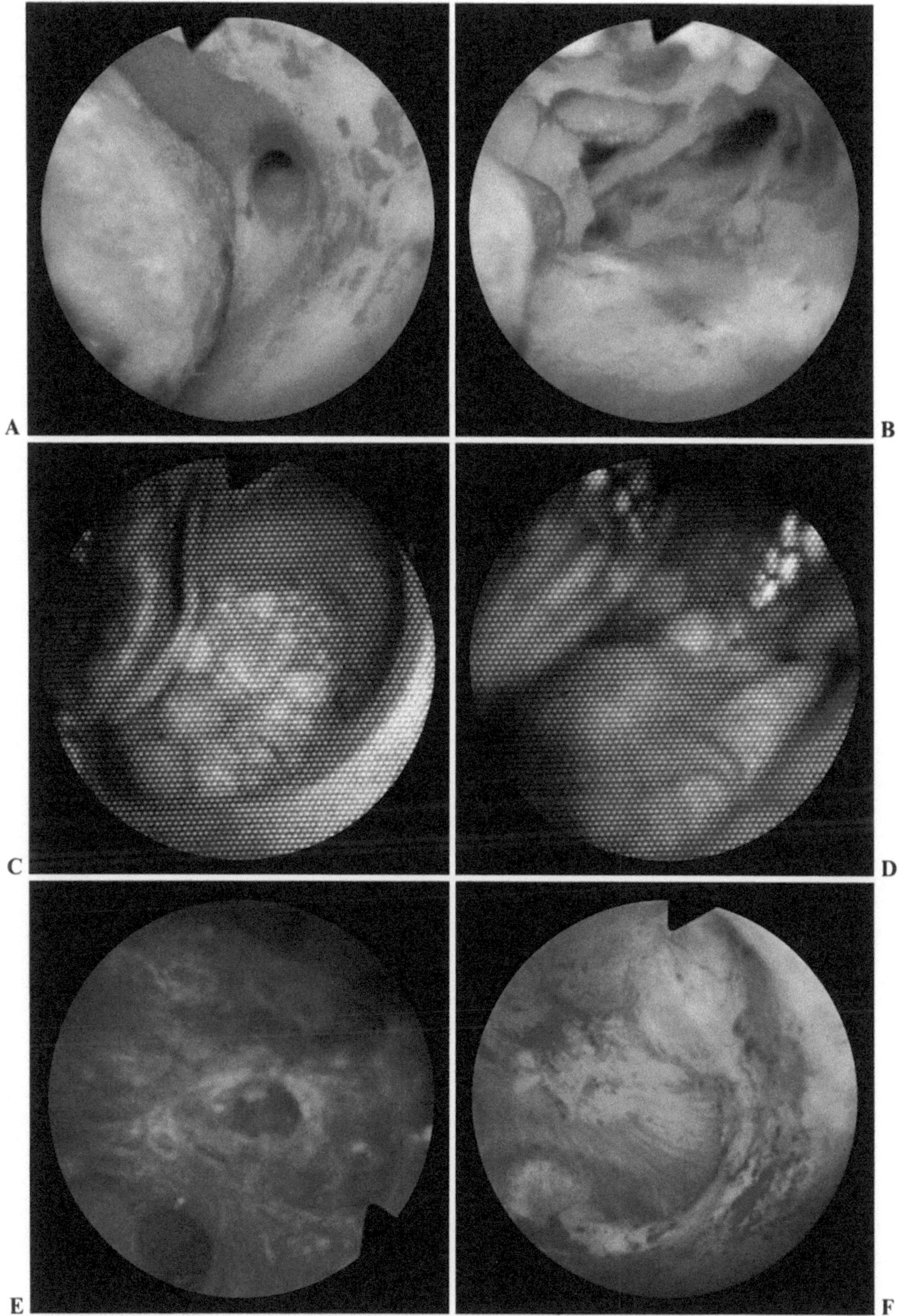

Plate II

G Numerous small calyceal stones in a horseshoe kidney

H Large recurrent pelvic stone (oxalate)

I After electrohydraulic disintegration the fragments are manipulated with the stone punch

K Large pelvic stone (Struvite) before disintegration. Ureter is blocked by a balloon catheter

L After the stone is disintegrated and the large fragments removed, many small pieces are still in the calyx

M After suction the calyx is clean, except for a tiny fragment (microsurgery!)

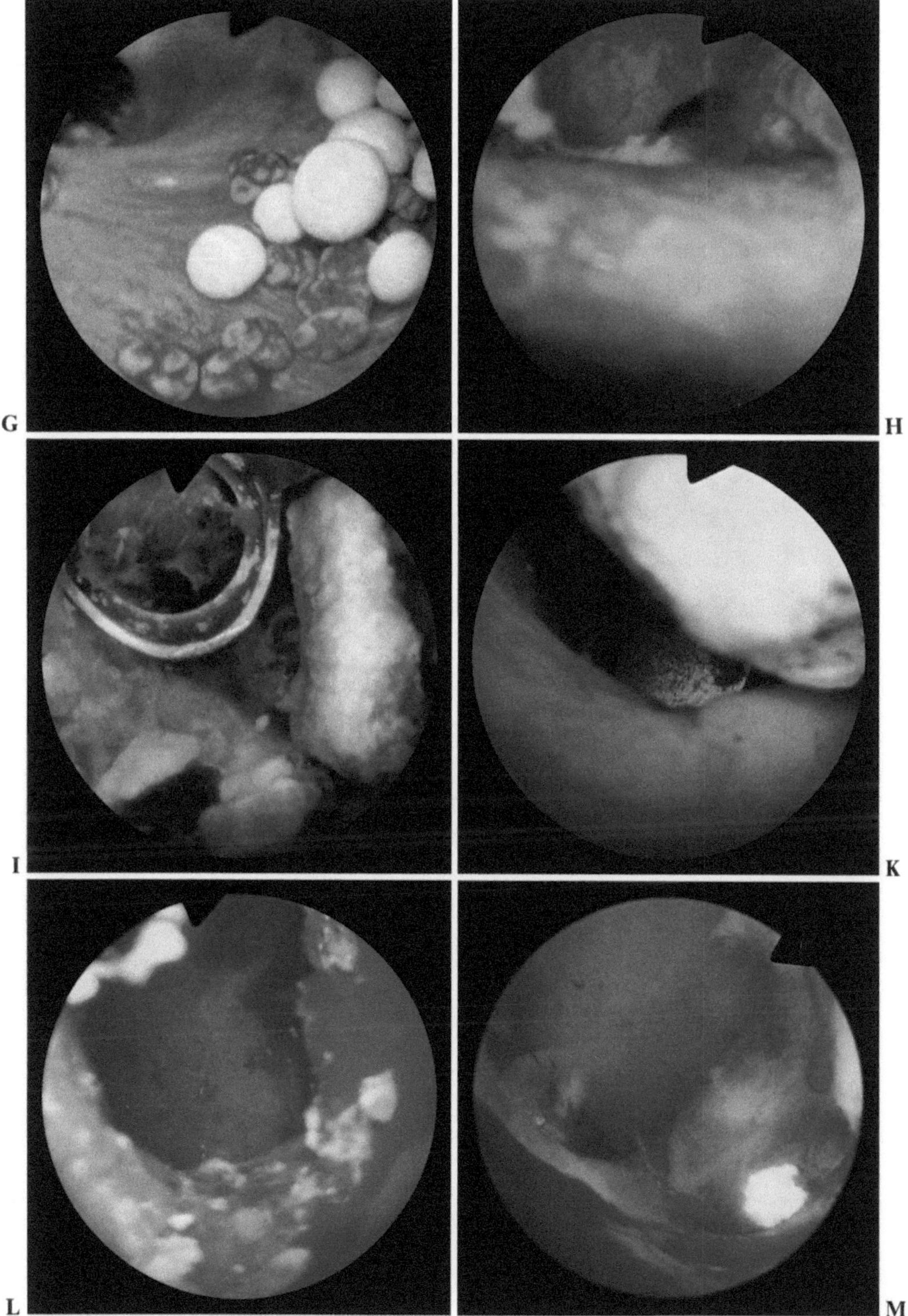
G
H
I
K
L
M

Plate III

N Electrohydraulic disintegration of a stone in the upper ureter via the flexible fiberscope (see also Fig. 47)

O Papillary renal tumor grade I (see also Fig. 62b)

P Base of the tumor after resection

Q Papillary tumor of the renal pelvis grade II before resection

R The tumor is macroscopically removed after it is resected and its base cauterized. The kidney is now treated locally with cytostatics through the nephrostomy catheter

S Marsupialization of a renal cyst. Below is a view of the renal pelvis. Above, the renal cyst with a black background. The thin wall, which for the most part is void of vessels, is resected with the resection loop in order to join the cyst to the renal pelvis (see also Fig. 63)

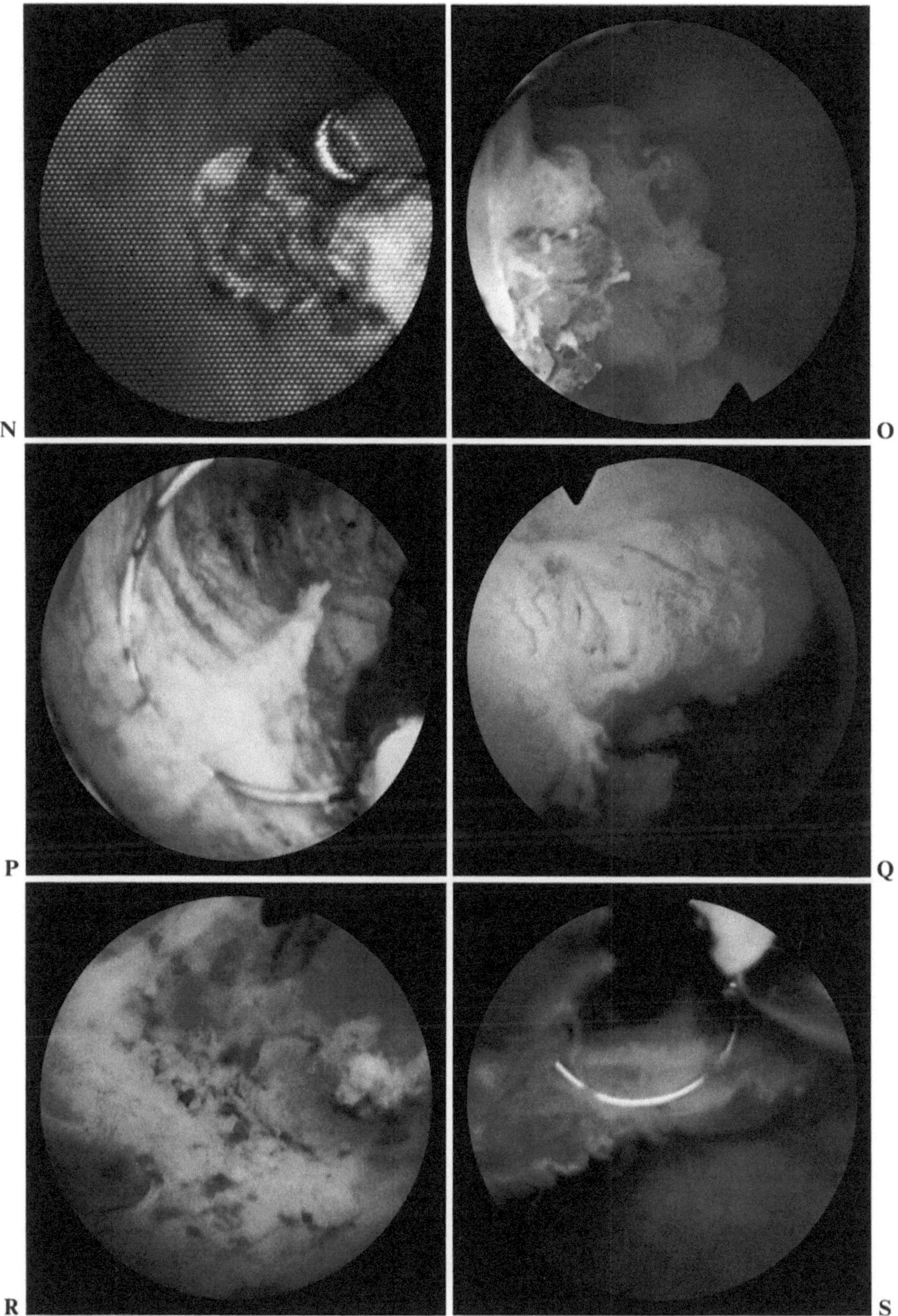

References

Alken P, Hutschenreiter, Günter R, Marberger M (1981) Percutaneous stone manipulation. J Urolog 125:463–466

Alken P (1981) Teleskopbourgieset zur perkutanen Nephrostomie. Akt Urolog 12:216–219

Fernström J, Johansson B (1976) Percutaneous nephrolithotomy. A new extraction technique. Scand J Urolog Nephrolog 10:257–259

Goodwin WE, Casey WC, Woolf W (1955) Percutaneous trocar (needle) nephrostomy in hydronephrosis. JAMA 157:891–893

Günther R, Alken P, Altwein JE (1979) Percutaneous nephrostomy using a fine needle-puncture set. Radiology 132:228–230

Korth K (1983) Perkutane Lithotrypsie mit einem neuen Dauerspül-Pyeloskop. Urolog A 22:219–221

Korth K (1983) A new percutaneous pyeloscope with permanent irrigation. British J of Urolog 31–33

Korth K (1983) The new percutaneous transrenal pyeloscope. Acta urol belg 51:484–486

Kurth KH, Hohenfellner R, Altwein JE (1977) Ultrasound litholapaxy of a staghorn calculus. J Urolog 117:242–243

Lutzeyer W, Pohlmann R, Terhorst B, Cichos M (1970) Die Zerstörung von Harnsteinen durch Ultraschall. I Experimentelle Untersuchungen. Urolog int 25:47–63

Wickham JEA, Miller R (1983) Percutaneous surgery of renal calculi. Churchill-Livingstone, London-Edinburgh

Subject Index

W. Mauermayer

Transurethral Surgery

With contributions by K. Fastenmeier,
G. Flachenecker, R. Hartung, W. Schütz
Translated from the German by A. Fiennes
Foreword by E. W. Goodwin

1983. 240 figures, 14 color plates. XXIX, 473 pages
ISBN 3-540-11869-1

Contents: Operating Facilities for Transurethral
Surgery. – Instruments and Their Care. – Preoperative
Requirements. – General Resection Technique
Cutting Methods and Techniques. – Special Resection
Technique. – Hemostatic Technique. – Transurethral
Bladder Surgery. – Special Resection Procedures
Around the Bladder Neck. – Litholapaxy. – The Zeiss
Loop and the Placement of Indwelling Ureteric Cathe-
ters. – Endoscopic Procedures in the Urethra. –
Urethral Dilation. – Postoperative Management. –
Learning and Teaching Transurethral Operative Tech-
nique. – Color Plates. – References. – Subject Index.

From the foreword:
"The present book, now in its English edition, is the
result of more than 30 years experience in transurethral surgery. During this time more than 10,000
patients were treated in Mauermayer's clinic by
various endoscopic operations. His unusual reservoir
of experience forms the basis for this book. It seems of
particular importance that surgical techniques are
described in a number of steps, since this enables even
a novice to understand the various procedures... He
also describes many tried and proven "clinical secrets",
which are illustrated by means of numerous outstan-
ding drawings. A number of excellent color illustra-
tions at the end of the book demonstrate his impres-
sive cystoscopic photography... I hope that this text-
book will reach a wide audience in the United States
and other English speaking countries where it deserves
a warm reception."   *Willard E. Goodwin*

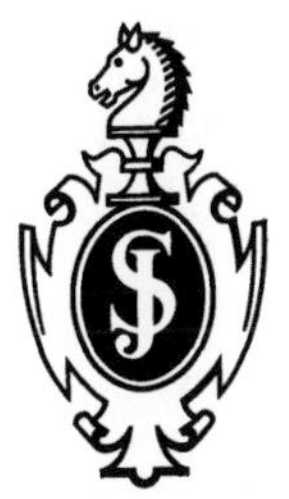

Springer-Verlag
Berlin
Heidelberg
New York
Tokyo

Disturbances in Male Fertility

By K. Bandhauer, G. Bartsch, D. M. de Kretser, A. Eshkol, J. Frick,
M. Glezerman, J. B. Kerr, B. Lunenfeld, W. Pöldinger, H. P. Rohr,
F. Scharfetter, P. D. Temple-Smith

Editors: K. Bandhauer, J. Frick

1982. 153 figures. XXIII, 454 pages. (Handbuch der Urologie/
Encyclopedia of Urology, Volume 16). ISBN 3-540-05279-8

Contents: Anatomical and Functional Aspects of the Male Repro-
ductive Organs. – Quantitative Morphology of the Prostate and
Epididymis. – Etiology of Fertility Disturbances in Man. – Male
Fertility Disorders-History and Clinical Examination. – Semen
Analysis. – Testicular Biopsy. – Radiologic Investigation of Male
Fertility Disorders. – Endocrine Evaluation of Male Fertility
Disorders. – Neurology of Male Fertility Disorders. – Immuno-
logic Causes of Male Fertility Disorders. – Treatment of Male
Infertility. – Operative Therapy of Male Infertility. – Artificial
Insemination and Semen Preservation. – Male Contraception. –
Impotence. – Functional Sexual Disorders in the Male. – Male
Climacteric? – Subject Index.

This volume provides urologists, andrologists, gynecologists,
dermatologists, and internists with modern, comprehensive des-
cription of the diagnosis and treatment of male infertility.

Central to the presentation is a consideration of the questions
relevant to clinical practice. The book also lays the foundation for
an understanding of the causes of male infertility with is detailed
account of the anatomy, physiology, pathophysiology, and functional of the testes and other glandular organs in the male reproductive tract. The major conceptual determinant is, however, the
complex of problems involved in male fertility disorders, ranging
from morphologic changes and endocrinologic, genetic, immunologic and vascular disturbances, to external and psychomatic
factors.

The contributors to this volume – each of them a leading specia-
list in his field – base their discussions on the current morphologic and functional knowledge of the various organs in the male
reproductive apparatus. Together they cover the following topics:

- etiology of fertility disturbances in men
- clinical aspects of semen analysis
- testicular biopsy
- radiologic examination of male infertility disorders
- endocrinologic and neurologic causes of male infertility
- immunologic problems in diagnosis and treatment
- artificial insemination and semen preservation
- impotence, the male climacteric, and functional sexual disorders.

This sythesis of morphology and function, of the principles of
spermiogenesis and the various factors affecting sperm formation
and maturation, as well as of the most important developments in
basic research and their clinical implications set **Disturbances in
Male Fertility** apart from all others in the field. The book includes
a critical evaluation of the relevant literature as well as a comprehensive bibliography.

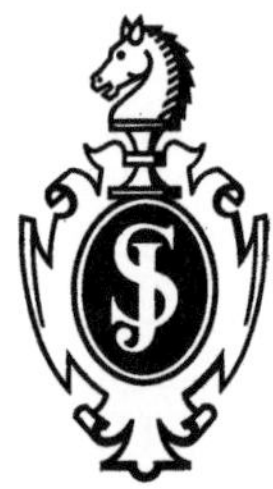

Springer-Verlag
Berlin
Heidelberg
New York
Tokyo

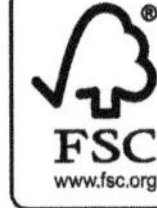

MIX
Papier aus verantwortungsvollen Quellen
Paper from responsible sources
FSC® C105338

If you have any concerns about our products,
you can contact us on
ProductSafety@springernature.com

In case Publisher is established outside the EU,
the EU authorized representative is:
Springer Nature Customer Service Center GmbH
Europaplatz 3, 69115 Heidelberg, Germany

Printed by Libri Plureos GmbH
in Hamburg, Germany